Sensory Systems I

Readings from the *Encyclopedia of Neuroscience*

Abnormal States of Brain and Mind
Selected and with an Introduction by J. Allan Hobson

Comparative Neuroscience and Neurobiology
Selected and with an Introduction by Louis N. Irwin

Learning and Memory
Selected and with an Introduction by Richard F. Thompson

Sensory Systems I: Vision and Visual Systems
Selected and with an Introduction by Richard Held

Sensory Systems II: Senses Other than Vision
Selected and with an Introduction by Jeremy Wolfe

Speech and Language
Selected and with an Introduction by Doreen Kimura

States of Brain and Mind
Selected and with an Introduction by J. Allan Hobson

Readings from the
Encyclopedia of Neuroscience

Sensory Systems I
Vision and Visual Systems

Selected and with an Introduction by
Richard Held

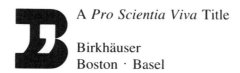

A *Pro Scientia Viva* Title

Birkhäuser
Boston · Basel

Library of Congress Cataloging-in-Publication Data
Sensory systems I.
    (Readings from the Encyclopedia of neuroscience)
    ''A Pro scientia viva title.''
    Bibliography: p.
    1. Vision.   2. Eye—Diseases and defects.
I. Held, Richard.   II. Series.
QP475.S47   1988   591.1′823   88-19364

CIP-Titelaufnahme der Deutschen Bibliothek
Readings from the Encyclopedia of neuroscience.—Boston ;
Basel : Birkhäuser.
    (A pro scientia viva title)
Sensory systems.
    1. Vision and visual systems.—1988
Sensory systems.—Boston ; Basel : Birkhäuser.
    (Readings from the Encyclopedia of neuroscience)
    (A pro scientia viva title)
1. Vision and visual systems / selected and with an introd. by
    Richard Held.—1988
    ISBN 3-7643-3395-2 (Basel) brosch.
    ISBN 0-8176-3395-2 (Boston) brosch.
NE: Held, Richard [Hrsg.]

Printed and bound by Edwards Brothers Incorporated, Ann Arbor, Michigan.
Printed in the United States of America.

9 8 7 6 5 4 3 2 1

ISBN 0-8176-3395-2
ISBN 3-7643-3395-2

Series Preface

This series of books, "Readings from the *Encyclopedia of Neuroscience*," consists of collections of subject-clustered articles taken from the *Encyclopedia of Neuroscience*.

The *Encyclopedia of Neuroscience* is a reference source and compendium of more than 700 articles written by world authorities and covering all of neuroscience. We define neuroscience broadly as including all those fields that have as a primary goal the understanding of how the brain and nervous system work to mediate/control behavior, including the mental behavior of humans.

Those interested in specific aspects of the neurosciences, particular subject areas or specialties, can of course browse through the alphabetically arranged articles of the *Encyclopedia* or use its index to find the topics they wish to read. However, for those readers—students, specialists, or others—who will find it useful to have collections of subject-clustered articles from the *Encyclopedia*, we issue this series of "Readings" in paperback.

Students in neuroscience, psychology, medicine, biology, the mental health professions, and other disciplines will find that these collections provide concise summaries of cutting-edge research in rapidly advancing fields. The nonspecialist reader will find them useful summary statements of important neuroscience areas. Each collection was compiled, and includes an introductory essay, by an authority in that field.

George Adelman
Editor,
Encyclopedia of Neuroscience

Contents

Series Preface v

Introduction
Richard Held xi

Amblyopia: Dullness of Vision
Theodore Lawwill 1

Attention, Selective Visual
Shimon Ullman and Christof Koch 3

Blindness, Neural Prosthesis
G.S. Brindley 5

Blindsight, Residual Vision
Ernst Pöppel 6

Brightness
Lewis O. Harvey, Jr. 7

Colliculus, Superior
Peter H. Schiller 9

Color Vision
Nigel W. Daw 10

Color Vision, Deficiencies
Leo M. Hurvich 12

Color Vision and Retinex Theory
Edwin H. Land 14

Cone Photoreceptors, Color Specificities
Teruya Ohtsuka 19

Electroretinogram, Electroretinography
John C. Armington 21

Eye-Head Coordination
Emilio Bizzi 23

Fly, Visual System
Kuno Kirschfeld 25

Fly, Visually Induced Behavior
Werner Reichardt 27

Gaze, Control of
Reuben S. Gellman and Frederick A. Miles 30

Gase, Plasticity in the Control of
Frederick A. Miles and Reuben S. Gellman 31

Geniculate Body, Lateral
Pedro Pasik and Tauba Pasik 33

Imagery, Mental
Stephen M. Kosslyn 35

Nystagmus
Volker Henn 37

Oculomotor System, Mechanisms
Masao Ito 38

Optic Nerves, Optic Chiasm, and Optic Tracts
Christopher Walsh 41

Optic Tectum
David J. Ingle 44

Reading
Marcel Kinsbourne 46

Retina, Neurotransmitters
Dianna A. Redburn 48

Retina, Vertebrate
John E. Dowling 50

Retinal Ganglion Cells
Mark Wm. Dubin 53

Retinotectal Interactions
S.C. Sharma 55

Stereopsis, Binocular Perception
John P. Frisby 57

Strabismus: Ocular Malalignment
Theodore Lawwill 59

Striate Cortex
Peter H. Schiller 61

Texture Perception
Bela Julesz 63

Vision, Deprivation Studies
Nigel W. Daw 65

Vision, Extrageniculostriate
Tauba Pasik and Pedro Pasik 67

Vision, Visual Cortex, and Frequency Analysis
Daniel A. Pollen and James P. Gaska 69

Visual Adaptation, Dark, Light
John C. Armington 71

Visual Aftereffects
Jeremy M. Wolfe 74

Visual Cortex
Max Cynader 76

Visual Cortex, Extrastriate
David C. Van Essen 80

Visual Development, Infant
Richard Held 82

Visual Field
Ernst Pöppel 85

Visual Learning, Pattern and Form Perception: Central Mechanisms
Howard C. Hughes and James M. Sprague 88

Visual Motion Perception
Shimon Ullman 91

Visual Perception
Jeremy M. Wolfe 93

Visual System, Organization
John Allman 95

Visual System, Siamese Cats
Carla J. Shatz 99

Visual System Development, Invertebrates
Eduardo R. Macagno and Ian A. Meinertzhagen 103

Visual System Development, Plasticity
Paul Grobstein and Kao Liang Chow 107

Visual Transduction
Gordon L. Fain and Wayne L. Hubbell 110

Visual-Vestibular Interaction
Volker Henn 114

Contributors 117

Introduction

Having found the articles on vision in the *Encyclopedia of Neuroscience* useful myself, I was pleased to write a short introduction to this collection, which has been culled from the *Encyclopedia*. These are brief, informative papers, written by experts in the field, who have extracted the essence of recent vision research and presented the material in terms which will be broadly informative to students, but also provide enough hard data to satisfy the ready-reference needs of people in the field. The publisher and I believe that there is a significant number of readers who will appreciate the availability of these papers as a collection of readings, a convenient and valuable source for information in the field of vision and vision research.

Who are these readers? First there are students in neuroscience, medicine, and psychology who will find these succinct and up-to-date articles a good resource to supplement their more general textbooks. Second, there are vision scientists and practitioners (ophthalmologists, optometrists), who on occasion need a source for state-of-the-art information for areas with which they may be unfamiliar or may have lost touch. Third, there are the scientists, artists, and other professionals who have a passing interest in vision and need an occasional reference at the level of detail provided by an *Encyclopedia* article. And then there are always students of vision who can profit by the substance and perspective given by different writers on their own special topics. That experts in the field wrote these articles is reflected in their brevity as well as in their quality. Only a writer well versed in an area can extract its essence. These authors have done just that.

The study of vision has sometimes been called the royal road to an understanding of the brain and nervous system. This metaphor acknowledges the belief that we know most about this aspect of brain function. Furthermore, it implies that principled knowledge derived from study of the visual brain may apply to our understanding of other parts of the brain and their function. It may be useful to consider the reasons for this assessment. A vast amount of work on vision, using behavioral and psychophysical methods, has accumulated over the past century. Far more effort has gone into research on vision than on any other sense, including its nearest competitor—hearing. This knowledge provides a background of technique and quantitative data which has been applied to the study of the "visual" nervous system, the large amount of brain involved in some aspect of vision or visual processing. In suitable laboratory preparations, cells of the visual nervous system respond quite systematically to visual stimulation just as do whole organisms. Moreover, such stimulation is easily controlled and may range from gross changes in luminance to fine nuances of pattern and color. By these stimulation experiments at the cellular level, a vast amount of knowledge has been collected about the transmission and processing of information within the nervous system as a whole as well as the visual nervous system in particular. Neuronal activation by stimulation has also been used to delineate anatomical connections by the use of substances (cell stains, radioactive tracers, etc.) that selectively mark the most activated cells in the system. We now know a great deal about the anatomical "wiring diagram" of the visual brain, especially about the major pathways for transmission of information, and much has been discovered about the physiology of cells and their synaptic connections. And, finally, we have increasing insight into the process of development, which lays down the connections within the system and the deviations from normal development (plasticity) that occur under various anomalous conditions of rearing. (This latter knowledge of course has important bearing on certain pathologies of vision.)

I have used these considerations in selecting and organizing this set of ''Readings.'' Although the articles are arranged in alphabetic order, for ease of reference we have provided five subject categories under which the titles of the articles may be grouped:

I. Psychophysics and Behavior

Gaze, Control of
Gaze, Plasticity in the Control of
Nystagmus
Oculomotor System, Mechanisms
Eye-Hand Coordination
Visual-Vestibular Interaction
Fly, Visually Induced Behavior
Brightness
Visual Adaptation, Dark, Light
Color Vision, Deficiencies
Color Vision, Retinex Theory
Visual Field
Optic Tectum
Stereopsis, Binocular Perception
Visual Aftereffects
Visual Motion Perception
Texture Perception
Visual Development, Infant
Visual Perception
Vision, Extrageniculostriate
Visual Learning, Pattern and Form
    Perception: Central Mechanisms
Attention, Selective Visual
Imagery, Mental
Reading

II. Anatomy

Cone Photoreceptors, Color
    Specificities
Visual Transduction
Retina, Vertebrate
Fly, Visual System
Visual System Development,
    Invertebrates
Oculomotor System, Mechanisms
Optic Nerves, Optic Chiasm, and
    Optic Tracts
Optic Tectum
Colliculus, Superior
Geniculate Body, Lateral
Striate Cortex
Visual Cortex
Visual Field
Vision, Deprivation Studies
Visual System, Siamese Cats

Vision, Extrageniculostriate
Visual Cortex, Extrastriate
Visual System, Organization
Visual Learning, Pattern and Form
    Perception: Central Mechanisms

III. Physiology

Cone Receptors, Color Specificities
Visual Transduction
Retina, Neurotransmitters
Retinal Ganglion Cells
Retina, Vertebrate
Electroretinogram,
    Electroretinography
Fly, Visual System
Retinotectal Interactions
Visual-Vestibular Interaction
Visual Cortex
Visual Motion Perception
Color Vision
Amblyopia: Dullness of Vision
Vision, Visual Cortex, and
    Frequency Analysis
Attention, Selective Visual

IV. Development and Plasticity

Visual System Development,
    Invertebrates
Retinotectal Interactions
Visual System, Development,
    Plasticity
Vision, Deprivation Studies
Amblyopia: Dullness of Vision
Visual Development, Infant

V. Pathology

Electroretinogram,
    Electroretinography
Visual Field
Blindness, Neural Prosthesis
Visual Learning, Pattern and Form
    Perception: Central Mechanisms
Strabismus: Ocular Malalignment
Amblyopia: Dullness of Vision
Blindsight, Residual Vision
Reading

Finally, a word about trends that will influence future developments in visual neuroscience as well as future editions of the *Encyclopedia of Neuroscience*. Two major developments that are already suggested in a number of the articles in this collection concern 1) the increasing amount of research on the cellular and molecular processes in the visual nervous system, and 2) the increasing prevalence of sophisticated modeling of the computations that must be performed by the visual system. Each of these may well become a major theme in future neuroscience research and be reflected in future compendia of progress.

Richard Held
Professor of Psychology
Massachusetts Institute of Technology

Amblyopia: Dullness of Vision

Theodore Lawwill

Amblyopia means dullness of vision. This clinical term refers to conditions where there is a partial loss of vision. The loss may be from any cause. The dullness of vision is variously described depending upon the origin, but is most easily related to the inability to distinguish form, particularly forms of small size such as the letters on a visual acuity chart. Light sense is not significantly affected.

Amblyopia is named on the basis of its origin: for example, toxic amblyopia, nutritional amblyopia, hysterical amblyopia, and functional amblyopia. The term functional amblyopia suggests inhibition of visual input from one eye. This common type of amblyopia is characterized by poor vision in one eye that occurs in an otherwise normal eye and is secondary to the disuse or improper use of the eye during early life. Functional amblyopia includes strabismic, sensory deprivation, and anisometropic and other types of refractive amblyopia. The incidence of amblyopia in the adult population has been estimated to be between 2% and 4%.

Functional amblyopia and binocular vision

Binocular vision is dependent not only upon the mechanism for accurate motor alignment of the visual axes upon the object of regard but also upon the innate neural pathways that connect corresponding points from the two retinas to the same cells in the visual cortex. These pathways allow single cortical cells to respond to the retinal cells from the two eyes that represent the same specific visual direction. This built-in mechanism for fusing the images from the two eyes can be disrupted by anything that unbalances the input from the two eyes. When the eyes are unbalanced under binocular conditions, the input from the disadvantaged eye to the binocularly reponsive cortical cells is decreased. This process can continue to the point of anatomical modification where visual acuity in that eye is permanently reduced. This may be reversible by forced use of the disadvantaged eye if begun at an early enough age, i.e., during the critical period during which the visual system exhibits structural and functional plasticity. Occlusion of the better eye for a period of time can restore vision to the amblyopic eye, but a separate population of cortical cells may then respond to each eye. While both eyes may have adequate visual acuity, they may be used alternately without fusion of the images from the two eyes.

One common cause of visual imbalance between the two eyes is strabismus in which the two eyes do not both point at the object of regard. When one eye is chosen as the favored eye, the image from the nonfavored eye is suppressed, a useful adaptation to avoid double vision. However, constant suppression at a young age leads to a permanent monocular visual deficit, strabismic amblyopia. Another type of amblyopia occurs if the two eyes have significantly different refractive errors. In this case, it is impossible for an object to be clearly focused on the two retinas at the same time without optical correction. When one eye is chosen to focus all the time, anisometropic amblyopia can develop in the other. If a clear image is not available during the early years, normal visual acuity does not develop. The most profound type of functional amblyopia is sensory deprivation amblyopia. This occurs when no image is allowed to reach the eye while the opposite eye is used normally. This may occur in cases such as unilateral congenital cataract or a severely drooping eyelid that precludes use of that eye during infancy.

The accepted treatment for functional amblyopia is forced use of the nonpreferred eye. This is usually accomplished by taping closed, i.e., patching, the preferred eye. The effectiveness of this treatment depends on the age at which it is instituted and the severity of the amblyopia.

Critical period

While the critical period for the development and reversal of functional amblyopia in monkeys has been studied and is fairly well known, less is known about this period in human development. In general the earlier the imbalance and the longer time before treatment, the greater the deficit produced and the less reversible it is. Deprivation or imbalance of only a week or two in an infant less than one year of age can trigger a significant amblyopia, particularly if some mild imbalance continues. Likewise, amblyopia can be more readily reversed at this early age. If the child passes 4 years of age with less than 20/200 visual acuity in the amblyopic eye, it is unlikely that 20/20 visual acuity will ever be achieved in that eye, even with several years of constant patching. Even after initially successful treatment those conditions of imbalance which lead to amblyopia usually continue to exist and can cause the amblyopia to recur. The visual acuity attained at the age of 10 or 12 years is usually retained without further therapy.

Functional amblyopia has been studied as a clinical model. These studies and studies on animal models of binocular vision have led to significant neurophysiological and neuroanatomical discovery. The important early observations of physiologists and clinicians, tedious psychophysical studies, and the famous and exciting neurophysiological studies of Hubel and Weisel have opened up a field of research with many possibilities. One potential area of applied study is the critical period for the development and reversal of functional amblyopia in humans. Several investigators are applying the technique of preferential looking developed by Teller to this question. Since there are many genetic and somatic differences between the visual systems of those affected by amblyopia, the task of isolating the controlling factors and the time course of the plasticity of the human visual system is not an easy one. However, the information will be of clinical and scientific importance.

Further reading

von Noorden GK, Burian HM (1979): *Burian-von Noorden's Binocular Vision and Ocular Motility: Theory and Management of Strabismus*, 2nd ed. St. Louis: CV Mosby

Attention, Selective Visual

Shimon Ullman and Christof Koch

A number of psychophysical studies concerning the detection, localization, and recognition of objects in the visual field have suggested a two-stage theory of human visual perception. The first stage is the preattentive mode, in which simple features are processed rapidly and in parallel over the entire visual field. In the second, attentive mode, a specialized processing mode, usually called the *focus of attention*, is directed to particular locations in the visual field. Recent psychophysical and physiological studies have provided more direct evidence for this focus of attention. Studies in this area received new impetus when it was shown that this so-called selective attention process plays a fundamental role even in the early stages of visual information processing.

Psychophysical evidence

Psychophysical studies suggest that the focus of *vision* can be directed, either voluntarily or by manipulating the visual stimulus, to different spatial locations in the visual scene. Studies by A. Treisman and G. Gelade have shown that visual search for targets defined by a single feature occurs in parallel across a visual display, whereas search for a target defined by a conjunction of two features requires a serial, self-terminating scan through distracting items. Thus, a search for a single red target among green background elements proceeds in parallel, and detection time does not depend on the number of distracting items (the so-called pop-out effect). In contrast, when the target is, for example, a vertical red line segment among vertical green and horizontal red distractors, finding the combination red-vertical proceeds serially, and detection time increases linearly with the number of distractors. B. Julesz has obtained similar results with both search and texture discriminating tasks, and his studies suggest that attentional shifts to a new location require roughly 30 msec. In a study by M. Posner a target was presented to the left or right of fixation. If subjects correctly anticipated the location at which the target would appear using prior cueing (an arrow at fixation), then their reaction time to the target in both detection and identification tasks was consistently lower (without eye movements). For simple detection tasks, the gain in detection time for a target at 7° eccentricity was on the order of 30 msec. This and similar studies suggest that subjects are able to shift their *visual attention* in advance to the cued location.

Physiological evidence

Phenomena related to the selective processing of visual information have also been investigated physiologically in the awake monkey in a number of different visual areas of the brain: the superior colliculus, the posterior parietal lobe (area 7), the frontal eye fields, areas V1, V2, V4, MT, MST, the inferior temporal lobe, and the pulvinar.

In the superficial layers of the superior colliculus of the monkey, many cells were found by Wurtz and his colleagues to have an enhanced response to a stimulus when the monkey uses the stimulus as a target for a saccadic eye movement. This enhancement is not strictly sensory in the sense that it is not produced if the stimulus is not followed by a saccade. It also does not seem strictly associated with a motor response, since the temporal delay between the enhanced response and the saccade can vary considerably. The relation of the enhancement to eye movements and its absence when the saccade is replaced by other responses suggest, however, that this mechanism is specifically related to saccadic eye movement rather than to operations associated with the shifting of visual attention.

Similar enhancement that depends on saccade initiation to a visual target has also been described in the frontal eye fields and in prestriate cortex. An area that exhibits enhancement phenomena, but not exclusively to saccades, is area 7 of the posterior parietal lobe. Using a series of peripheral attention tasks in which the monkey signals the dimming of a peripheral stimulus without making an eye movement toward the stimulus, Bushnell, Goldberg, and Robinson found that half of all cells studied give an enhanced response to this task. The enhancement is spatially specific, as it occurs mainly if the dimming is detected within the receptive field of the recorded neuron, and it also occurs when the monkey makes a saccade or points his hand at the stimulus. On the basis of these and similar findings, it was suggested that mechanisms in area 7 are responsible for directing visual attention to selected stimuli.

Recent experiments in P. Schiller's laboratory demonstrate selective gating in V4. In this experiment the monkey was required to release a dial if it detected an agreement between tactile and visual stimuli (if the orientation of line grooves on a dial paralleled the orientation of a visually presented grating). While some cells responded to a specific visual cue independently of the tactile one, e.g., they always responded to a horizontal grating, some discharged only if there was no discrepancy in the orientations of the two patterns. It is unclear, however, whether this gating depends also on the location to be processed or only upon the nature of the task.

In a number of visual areas of the cortex, including V1, V2, and MT, enhanced responses associated with performing specific visual tasks were not found. It remains possible, however, that task-specific modulation will be observed when employing different visual tasks.

The notion of a processing focus that can be directed selectively to different locations in the visual field also receives support from computational studies by S. Ullman. Various computations that are useful in the recognition of shapes are facilitated if different computations can be applied selectively to particular regions in the image. Moreover, the need for a serial processing stage in visual information processing becomes apparent when one considers that the system is unlikely to assume multiple mechanisms for performing tasks, such as shape analysis and recognition, in parallel over the whole visual scene. Such an approach would quickly lead to a combinatorial explosion in terms of required computational resources.

Taken together, these psychophysical, physiological, and computational studies reinforce the two-stage theory of human visual perception. The first stage is the preattentive mode in which simple features such as local orientation, color, depth, and direction of motion are computed in parallel across the visual field. Subsequently, the second, attentive mode operates on these basic representations using a serial scanning mechanism.

Further reading

Haenny P, Maunsell J, Schiller P (1984): Cells in prelunate cortex alter response to visual stimuli of different behavioral significance. *Perception* 13:A7

Julesz B (1984): A brief outline of the texton theory of human vision. *Trend Neurosci* 7:41–48

Koch C, Ullman S (1985): Shifts in selective visual attention: Towards the underlying neural circuitry. *Human Neurobiol* 4:219–227

Posner MI (1980): Orienting of attention. *Q J Exp Psychol* 32:3–25

Treisman A, Gelade G (1980): A feature integration theory of attention. *Cog Psychol* 12:97–136

Ullman S (1984): Visual routines. *Cognition* 18:97–159

Wurtz RH, Goldberg ME, Robinson DL (1982): Brain mechanisms of visual attention. *Sci Am* 246(6):124–135

Blindness, Neural Prosthesis

G.S. Brindley

During and soon after World War I, German neurosurgeons discovered that if a point on the cerebral cortex near the posterior pole of either cerebral hemisphere was stimulated electrically during an intracranial operation done under local anesthesia, the patient reported seeing a spot of light. The spot was small and lay in the half of the visual field opposite to the hemisphere that was stimulated. The position of the light varied with the part of the hemisphere stimulated. One of these early patients had been hemianopic for 8 years. Electrical stimulation caused him to see lights in the blind half of his field of vision.

It was natural to hope from these facts that if one designed an implant that allowed stimulation through any of a large number of electrodes placed near the posterior pole of each cerebral hemisphere, one could enable a blind person to see. Three devices intended for this purpose have been designed and implanted in England (in 1967, 1972, and 1982) and three in the United States (all between 1973 and 1975). All six implants have had limited success. The blind patients could be caused to see spots of light at places in the visual field that were fairly constant from minute to minute and from week to week. If stimulation was done through several electrodes at the same time, predictable patterns of spots of light could be built up. One English patient and one American patient could read braille by means of their implants, but not as fast or as accurately as they could read it with their fingers. None of the implants has been of significant practical use.

The places on the cortex where stimulation consistently causes the patient to see spots of light lie in cortical areas 17 and 18 of Brodmann (striate and parastriate). The sensations from 18 are very similar to those from 17. Animal experiments would lead one to expect a regular (though distorted) map of each visual half-field on the opposite area 17, and a second such map on area 18, but the observations on blind patients with implants do not easily fit this expectation.

Stimulation of area 19 during neurosurgical operations has sometimes caused visual sensations, but these have usually been complex, not pointlike. Electrodes on area 19 have not yet been used in visual prosthetic implants.

The English implants were driven by radio power from transmitters mounted in a hat. The American implants had wires running through the skin, either directly or in a Pyrolite carbon pedestal. All the implants, English or American, were in principle capable of being driven from a television camera. However, it may be more practical to use a camera with a matrix of photocells in its image plane, the photocells being connected so that signals can be obtained from all of them simultaneously.

Great improvements in visual prosthetic implants are possible, and the English group that designed the first, second, and sixth implants is still working on the engineering problems. However, these problems are substantial, and the benefit that blind people can expect when they are solved is not necessarily very great. Electrical stimulation inactivates the local analyzing mechanisms of the cortical areas stimulated. Partly for this reason, the spatial resolving power of the brain for such stimulation is poor, and it seems unlikely that more than 1000 different sites of stimulation can usefully be discriminated. A television screen contains roughly 40,000 separately controllable points, and each human optic nerve about a million nerve fibers, so the quality of vision with a visual prosthetic implant will be poor, if the physiological limitation to about 1000 points that now seems probable proves in the end to be correct.

Observations on the first six implants strongly suggest that the useful introduction of color into what the patient sees will not be possible. Some of the patients do indeed see colored spots, but the colors are not stable from day to day, and it is not possible to vary them independently of the position and intensity.

If visual prosthetic implants are to have an application in the future, it may be restricted to the small minority of blind people who, on becoming blind as adults, remain strongly motivated to read and wish to read any typeface and handwriting, so that character-recognizing machines will not meet their needs. People who are born blind or lose their sight as children and wish to read handwriting can do so with the Optacon, which translates optical images into patterns that can be read with the fingers and can be used with any typeface, or with good handwriting. However, people who lose their sight as adults rarely succeed in becoming efficient Optacon users. A thousand-point visual prosthetic implant, if a good one can be designed, may meet the special needs of those among them who need to read manuscript and unusual type. Such an implant will probably also be useful for getting about, but it will be no better than a guide dog for this purpose.

Further reading

Brindley GS (1982): Effects of electrical stimulation of the visual cortex. *Human Neurobiol* 1:281–283

Blindsight, Residual Vision

Ernst Pöppel

A lesion within the geniculostriatal projection of the visual system produces a scotoma i.e., an area of blindness in a corresponding region of the visual field. Until recently, such blindness, determined by visual field measurement or perimetry, has been considered absolute. However, observations with nonhuman primates involving experimental ablation of striate cortex or parts of it have shown that visual information can still be processed in regions of the visual field that are blind. Such animals are observed to look toward targets that, because of their brain lesion, they are not supposed to see. On the basis of such evidence, the visual capacities of human subjects have been tested using nonverbal techniques. Most of the human subjects, i.e., patients that have suffered a lesion within the geniculostriatal projection system, can demonstrate some residual vision. They are able to look toward unseen targets within their scotoma.

Because these patients appear to be blind on the basis of visual field measurements, but can still process visual information, the term blindsight is used for their residual vision. The fact that patients are able to look toward targets they cannot see implies that the oculomotor system has access to visual stimuli within the scotoma. But other visual functions have also been demonstrated in such patients. For example, the presence or absence of visual targets can be indicated by mere guessing without moving the eyes. This kind of residual vision has been demonstrated using a signal detection paradigm. Signal detection techniques show that blindsight cannot be an artifact due to scattered light, because the presentation of a visual target at the natural blind spot within or outside the cortical scotoma does not result in residual vision. If scattered light were responsible for residual vision, the blind spot should also be sensitive to visual stimulation. The signal detection paradigm has also shown that different colors can be discriminated that are presented within the scotoma; other studies had shown positive evidence of residual pattern discrimination.

For some researchers the term blindsight implies that residual vision is based on a specific central projection of the retina, i.e., the pathway from the retina via the superior colliculus and the pulvinar complex of the thalamus to the extrastriate cortex. But such a conclusion may be premature. There are at least four different pathways that might mediate residual visual function; furthermore, it appears reasonable to assume that different residual functions are mediated by different pathways.

Evidence from experiments with nonhuman primates suggests that the guidance of saccadic eye movements toward targets within a scotoma is based on the representation of the visual field in the superior colliculus. It is, however, unlikely that this pathway is also responsible for residual color discrimination. In this case the projection from the retina to lateral geniculate nucleus and from there to the extrastriate cortex could be responsible. But also a direct projection from the retina to the pulvinar complex and then to extrastriate cortex could do the job. Perhaps, these pathways also account for residual pattern discrimination. But in this case the projection via the superior colliculus to the extrastriate cortex has also been suggested. Simple detection could also be mediated by either pathway, but a third anatomical possibility should not be neglected. It could well be that the striate cortex itself, although lesioned, is responsible for residual functions. An area of blindness in the visual field that has been determined by perimetry does not necessarily mean that there is no structural basis at all left to process visual information. Even a severely damaged striate cortex might still process visual information. This, however, might only be demonstrable by sensitive psychophysical techniques. The level of processing can be considered to be too low to result in a conscious representation of the stimulus.

As studies on blindsight have important implications for the understanding of the structural basis of human vision, it is necessary to stress the limitations of structural interpretations. What can be said, however, is that blindsight is a genuine phenomenon.

Further reading

Campion J, Latto R, Smith YM (1983): Is blindsight due to scattered light, spared cortex and near threshold effects? *Behav Brain Sci* 6:423–486

Pöppel E, Held R, Frost D (1973): Residual visual function after brain wounds involving the central visual pathways in man. *Nature* 243:295–296

Stoerig P, Hübner M, Pöppel E (1985): Signal detection analysis of residual vision in a field defect due to a post-geniculate lesion. *Neuropsychologia*, 23:589–599

Weiskrantz L, Warrington EK, Sanders MD, Marshall J (1974): Visual capacity in the hemianopic field following a restricted occipital ablation. *Brain* 97:709–723

Zihl, T (1980): 'Blindsight': improvement of visually guided eye movements by systematic practice in patients with cerebral blindness. *Neuropsychologia* 18:71–77

Brightness

Lewis O. Harvey, Jr.

Brightness is a psychological dimension that permits visual stimuli to be ordered from dark to light. Although brightness is related to the physical intensity of light, the relationship is complex, involving spatial and temporal interactions. Some authors use the term brightness to describe light sources and surfaces viewed in isolation, and the term lightness or whiteness to describe surfaces that are seen as part of objects and are viewed in relationship to other surfaces and objects. This distinction is not made here.

Basic brightness relationships

The physical intensity of light is expressed in luminance units of candela/square meter. The visual system operates in light intensities from about 10^{-6} to 10^{+6} cd/m^2, a range of 10^{+12} to 1. This tremendous range is mediated by two separate systems: scotopic vision, mediated by a single type of rod photoreceptor, and photopic vision, mediated by three (in normal trichromatic vision, at least) cone receptors. Scotopic vision operates from 10^{-6} to 10^{-2} cd/m^2; photopic vision from 10^{-2} to 10^{+6} (light of the full moon to bright sunlight). The ability to detect differences in brightness between a target and a larger background can be expressed in terms of the increment or decrement in luminance (Δ L) required for some constant level of detection performance (e.g., 75% correct). The ratio of Δ L to the background luminance L is called the Weber fraction. This fraction is a function of the exposure duration of the target, the size of the target, and the background luminance itself. The Weber fraction can be as high as 200 at very low scotopic luminances and steadily decrease as luminance is increased up to low photopic levels (10 cd/m^2). The Weber fraction stays constant (Weber's law) at higher photopic luminances, increasing slightly again at the upper limit of photopic vision. The value of the Weber fraction at any given luminance level depends reciprocally on the size of the stimulus and its exposure duration:

$$\frac{\Delta L}{L} \times \text{time} = k \qquad \text{Bloch's law (exposure duration)}$$

$$\frac{\Delta L}{L} \times \text{area} = k \qquad \text{Ricco's law (for small areas)}$$

$$\frac{\Delta L}{L} \times \text{area}^{0.5} = k \qquad \text{Piper's law (for larger areas)}$$

Bloch's law is only valid for exposures less than a critical duration. The critical duration is about 100 msec for low scotopic level of light and reduces to about 30 msec at higher photopic levels. Ricco's law holds for small stimuli (less than 10 min arc in diameter). Piper's law is a better description for larger areas.

Psychophysical scaling is used to develop number scales that represent the magnitude of the psychological experience of brightness. Various methods of measurement agree that the relationship between the psychological dimension of brightness and the physical dimension of luminance is nonlinear. An approximation to this relationship is given by the Stevens power relationship:

$$\text{brightness A} \times \text{L}^{\text{B}}$$

The value for the exponent B is usually given as 0.33, but it depends on target size and other viewing conditions. A specific scale of brightness based on the *Bril* unit was proposed by Hanes in 1949 but has not come into wide usage.

Brightness constancy

When viewing normal visual scenes containing a wide range of objects having different reflectances, the perceptual impression of the brightness of the surfaces corresponds more to the constant reflectance characteristics of the surface than to the luminance of the surface. This brightness constancy effect means that a white piece of paper (with reflectance of 0.75, for example) appears white in relatively dim light and in relatively bright light. Black ink printed on the white paper (reflectance of about 0.05) appears black under both lighting conditions, even though the black ink has a higher luminance when viewed in bright light than does the white paper viewed in dim light. Brightness of surfaces depends more on the ratios of luminances than on the absolute luminance values themselves. A surface having a particular luminance gets its brightness by being perceived in relation to the luminances of the surfaces around it in the visual scene. Without knowledge of the luminances of the other surfaces, it is not possible to predict the brightness of a particular luminance value: It could appear as any brightness from black to white. The ratio of luminances which under these conditions appear white and black is about 200:1; luminances greater than this level would appear self-luminous, not white; luminances less than the lower value appear no blacker than black.

Brightness constancy is not perfect; the brightness of surfaces shifts somewhat with increases in luminance, even though the luminance ratios remain constant. As overall illumination is increased by only a factor of 10 from low photopic levels, the brightness of surfaces shift in two opposite directions: whites become whiter and blacks blacker. The perceptual range between black and white increases by a factor of 1.4 when illumination increases by a factor of 10.

Brightness contrast

The brightness of a surface can be greatly modified by spatially adjacent surfaces. A gray area of fixed luminance will appear darker when surrounded by a white area than by a black area. This effect is asymmetrical: the white surrounding field makes the gray very much blacker while the darker surround only makes the gray a little whiter. The surrounding field (also called the inducing field) can be present simultaneously (simultaneous brightness contrast) or sequentially (metacontrast), but in the latter case the inducing field must be within approximately 200 msec of the test field for it to influence the brightness of that field. These contrast effects, because they occur over relatively large areas of the visual fields, are global effects. An interesting start at development of a model of global processing able to represent the complexities of brightness perception is that of Grossberg and Mingolla. This model contains nonlinear dynamic networks that segment the visual world in at least two ways: boundary contours and feature contours.

Other contrast effects are more local in nature. Mach bands, which enhance borders between areas of different luminances, and Hermann grid illusions, illusory dark spots at the intersections of a grid of white lines, are examples. These effects have been attributed to the center-surround organization of retinal ganglion cell receptive fields.

Temporal effects on brightness

Bloch's law implies a summation of energy up to the critical duration to create a specific brightness. Bloch's law applies to stimuli that are just barely detectable. With suprathreshold stimuli, the relationship between brightness and exposure duration is both nonlinear and nonmonotonic. Certain presentation times or rates of flickering presentation give an enhancement of brightness (Broca-Sulzer effect). The flicker frequency that gives the maximum brightness enhancement varies with luminance level but is in the range from 2 to 8 Hz.

Brightness is a psychological quantity that has a complex dependency on the luminance, spatial, and temporal characteristics of stimuli and on interactions with other stimuli. The basic relationship between brightness and luminance is a nonlinear power function. Spatial interactions are both local and global. The local interactions seem to be a consequence of neural organization at the level of the retinal ganglion cell. Plausible neural structures for global brightness processing and widely accepted neural codes representing brightness are yet to be determined.

Acknowledgments

This article was prepared while the author was Visiting Professor at the Institute for Medical Psychology, Ludwig-Maximilian University, Munich, as recipient of a fellowship from the Alexander von Humboldt Foundation, Bonn, Federal Republic of Germany. The kind and generous support of the foundation, the Institute, and Professors E. Pöppel and I. Rentschler is gratefully acknowledged.

Further reading

Cornsweet TN (1970): *Visual Perception*. New York: Academic Press

Grossberg S, Mingolla E (1985): Neural dynamics of perceptual grouping: Textures, boundaries, and emergent segmentations. *Percept Psychophys* 38:141–171

Hanes RM (1949): A scale of subjective brightness. *J Exp Psychol* 39:438–452

Hurvich LM, Jameson D (1966): *The Perception of Brightness and Darkness*. Boston: Allyn & Bacon

Judd DB (1951): Basic correlates of the visual stimulus. In: *Handbook of Experimental Psychology*, Stevens SS, ed. New York: John Wiley & Sons

Le Grand Y (1957): *Light, Colour, and Vision*, Hunt RWG, Walsh JWT, Hunt FRW, trans. London: Chapman and Hall

Colliculus, Superior

Peter H. Schiller

The superior colliculus is a laminated structure on the roof of the midbrain. In fish, amphibians, and reptiles, the superior colliculus is the center for analysis of visual information and sensorimotor integration. In higher mammals, as a result of the elaboration of the geniculocortical system, much of this analysis has been relegated to visual cortex, the volume of which far exceeds that of the colliculus. In the rhesus monkey, whose superior colliculus has been extensively studied, this ovoid structure is about the size of a pea, measuring approximately 6 mm in diameter and 2–3 mm in thickness.

The superficial layers of the superior colliculus are concerned exclusively with vision. This region receives input from both the retina and the visual cortex, and sends projections to the pulvinar and the nucleus parabigemini. The visual field is arranged in an orderly, topographic fashion on the surface of the colliculus. Each single cell is sensitive to a small region of the visual field, the cell's receptive field. In fish, amphibians, and reptiles, the receptive field properties of single cells can be complex. Cells may respond selectively to the orientation of line segments and the direction of stimulus movement. The structural organization of the colliculus matches this complexity, with many laminae and numerous cell types, some of which show considerable interlaminar interaction. By contrast, in higher mammals collicular organization is less elaborate. There are fewer laminae, the receptive field organization is simpler, and there appears to be less interaction among the laminae. In the rhesus monkey direction and orientation specificities are mostly absent. Cells respond preferentially to small stimuli and are not selective for other stimulus dimensions.

The deeper layers of the mammalian superior colliculus receive inputs from a large number of cortical and subcortical areas. The major outputs of these laminae are to those deeper regions of the midbrain and the brain stem that are concerned with the generation of eye movements. The response properties of single cells in this region differ from the superficial layers in three respects: (1) Some cells can be activated not only by visual, but also by somatosensory and auditory stimuli; (2) cells become progressively less responsive when stimuli are presented repeatedly; and (3) many cells respond vigorously prior to saccadic eye movements. Each eye-movement-related cell discharges in association with a small range of saccade sizes and directions. Eye movement cells are arranged in an orderly manner, forming a motor map in the colliculus. In the anterior regions of the colliculus these cells discharge prior to small saccades, in the posterior regions prior to large ones, in the medial portions prior to upward, and in the lateral portions to downward ones. The motor map appears to be in register with the sensory map, which in the anterior regions of the colliculus represents central vision, in the posterior regions peripheral vision, in the medial regions the upper, and in the lateral regions the lower visual field. Electrical stimulation of the intermediate and deep layers of the superior colliculus elicits saccadic eye movements at very low current levels: the size and direction of *eye movements* elicited depend on which portion of the structure is stimulated and are largely independent of the initial position of the eye in orbit. The size and direction of stimulation-elicited saccades can be predicted on the basis of the activity of eye movement neurons in the stimulated area. The computational processes involved in the generation of saccadic eye movements utilize both retinal error and eye position signals. Both of these signals have been shown to be available at the level of the superior colliculus.

The generation of saccadic eye movements involves both excitatory and inhibitory processes. The cortical input to the colliculus appears to be mostly excitatory, while inputs from the substantia nigra are inhibitory. The two colliculi interconnect extensively, and this connection also appears to be inhibitory. These observations suggest that the generation of saccadic eye movements by the superior colliculus involves not only excitatory but also disinhibitory processes. The complexity of cortical and subcortical interactions for the generation of orientation and eye movement is highlighted by the observation in the cat that deficits in visually guided locomotion, induced by large cortical lesions, can be reversed by sectioning the commissures connecting the left and right superior colliculi. This finding suggests that in the cat the colliculi are capable of performing significant visual analysis for orientation provided intercollicular inhibition is blocked.

Destruction of the superior colliculus in submammalian species causes serious deficits in vision and orientation. In primates the deficit is less pronounced, typically resulting in a moderate decrease in the frequency, velocity, and accuracy of saccadic eye movements. The restricted nature of these deficits appears to be due to the fact that a second pathway involving the frontal eye fields of the cortex contributes to the control of visually guided saccadic eye movements. When both the superior colliculi and the frontal eye fields are destroyed, monkeys can no longer make visually guided saccades.

Further reading

Schiller PH (1984): The superior colliculus and visual function. In: *Handbook of Physiology, Vol 3, part 1*. Darian-Smith I, ed. Bethesda: American Physiological Society

Color Vision

Nigel W. Daw

There are two aspects to color vision: the variety of wavelengths that can be distinguished, which is determined by the receptors in the retina and their spectral sensitivities, and the perception of color, which is determined by the neural connections within the visual system.

There are two classes of receptor in the retina, rods and cones. The receptors in the human retina that are responsible for color vision are the cones. Since there are three types of cones, long-wave, medium-wave, and short-wave absorbing cones, humans are called trichromats. Strictly speaking humans are tetrachromats, since they also have rod receptors, but in central vision the rods are absent, and in moderately bright daylight the rods are saturated, so that only the cones are active.

The number of receptors in other species varies. Goldfish are also trichromats, with pigments displaced toward longer wavelengths compared to the human. Cats have three types of receptor, but their retina is dominated by one of them. Ground squirrels are dichromats. Birds and turtles have colored oil droplets in front of their receptors, increasing the variety of spectral sensitivities so that they may effectively have more than three types of receptor. Macaque monkey receptors are very like the human.

In all species of animal that have so far been investigated, receptors converge onto opponent color cells, and opponent color cells converge at a higher level of the system onto double opponent cells. An opponent color cell is one that has an excitatory input from one type of receptor and an inhibitory input from another. For example, one type of opponent color cell is excited by long-wave receptors and inhibited by medium-wave receptors. These cells give an ON response to long-wave light, and an OFF response to medium-wave light (their firing rate is increased by long-wave light and decreased by medium-wave light, and a burst of action potentials occurs when the medium-wave light is turned off). They respond very little to white light, which is absorbed by both long-wave and medium-wave receptors, thus providing both excitatory and inhibitory input to the cell, summing up to little change in the membrane potential of the cell.

The response of opponent color cells corresponds, in a sense, to the phenomenon of successive color contrast. In the example given here, the cell will respond when white light is turned off and long-wave light is turned on. It will also respond when medium-wave light is turned off and white light is turned on. These two stimuli are equivalent stimuli to the cell, analogous to the common experience that staring at red light and then looking at a white card leads to a complementary colored green afterimage.

There must be a variety of opponent color cells. Given Hering's theory of opponent colors, one would predict that ON red OFF green, OFF red ON green, ON yellow OFF blue, and OFF yellow ON blue varieties should exist. Present

data indicate that this is probably the case, although the precise details have not been fully worked out.

Opponent color cells converge onto double opponent cells (Fig. 1). Double opponent cells are cells that are opponent for both color and space. Their receptive fields have a center-surround organization. The example shown in Figure 1 gives ON responses to long-wave light and OFF responses to medium-wave light illuminating the center of its receptive field. In the periphery of its receptive field, the responses are OFF to long-wave light and ON to medium-wave light. Such a cell responds only to color contrasts. Uniform long-wave light, uniform medium-wave light, white light in the center of the receptive field, and white light in the periphery of the receptive field all give a combination of excitatory and inhibitory inputs that cancel each other out and result in very little response from the cell. The largest excitatory response comes from long-wave light in the center of the receptive field and medium-wave light in the periphery. The largest inhibitory response comes from medium-wave light in the center of the receptive field and long-wave light in the periphery.

The response of double opponent cells explains the phenomenon of simultaneous color contrast. Consider the cell illustrated in Figure 1. A white or gray spot in a medium-wave surround will excite the double-opponent cell, and so will a long-wave spot in a white or gray surround. These stimuli are equivalent stimuli for the cell, corresponding to the perception that a white or gray spot in a green surround appears reddish.

Opponent color cells and double opponent cells have been investigated in three species: goldfish, ground squirrel, and macaque monkey. The hierarchy of cell types (receptors converging onto opponent color cells, which in turn converge onto opponent color cells) is the same in all three species, but the anatomical level at which the cells are found differs. In goldfish, horizontal and bipolar cells in the retina are opponent color. Some bipolar cells may be double opponent, but the level at which double opponent cells are found extensively is the ganglion cell level. In ground squirrel, ganglion cells are opponent color. The retina projects to the lateral geniculate body where double opponent cells are found. In macaque monkey, ganglion cells and lateral geniculate cells are opponent color. Double opponent cells are not found until one reaches the next level of the system, the visual cortex.

Perception of color is a complicated process that involves not only the wavelengths of light coming from the object looked at, but also the wavelengths of light coming from all the objects around it. In general, the color of an object is correlated much more closely with its reflectance, which is a physical property of the object, than with the wavelengths reflected from it, which depend on the wavelengths falling on the object as well as the reflectance of the object. That is why objects do not change color when moved from one envi-

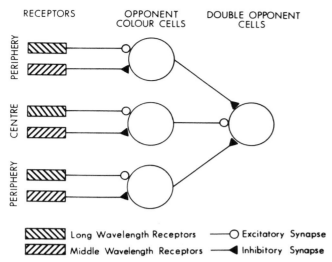

RECEPTORS   OPPONENT COLOUR CELLS   DOUBLE OPPONENT CELLS

▨ Long Wavelength Receptors   ──○ Excitatory Synapse
▨ Middle Wavelength Receptors   ──◀ Inhibitory Synapse

Figure 1. First three stages in the organization of color vision. Receptors synapse onto opponent color cells, which in this example would be excited by long wavelengths and inhibited by medium wavelengths. Opponent color cells synapse onto double opponent cells, which in this example would be excited by long wavelengths and inhibited by medium wavelengths in the center of their receptive fields, and excited by medium wavelengths and inhibited by long wavelengths in the periphery of their receptive fields.

ronment to another—a phenomenon called object color constancy.

The physiological mechanisms involved in object color constancy are still being worked out in experiments on the macaque monkey, which has color vision close to that of the human. The anatomical pathway for processing color information in this species involves projections from the retina to the lateral geniculate body, then to primary visual cortex (V1). In primary visual cortex there are clusters of cells called blobs, dealing particularly with color vision. Primary visual cortex is interconnected with secondary visual cortex (V2) which in turn is interconnected to another area of visual cortex (V4) that deals particularly with color. Secondary visual cortex is subdivided into areas that show up as thick and thin stripes with staining for cytochrome oxidase. The blobs in V1 project to the thin stripes in V2, which project to V4. In summary, there are now at least seven anatomical levels known in the processing of color vision: receptors, bipolar cells and ganglion cells in the retina, cells in the lateral geniculate, blobs in V1, thin stripes in V2, and V4. Other levels will almost certainly be discovered: for example, the areas around the blobs in V1 also have color properties, as do the cells in the blobs.

While the physiology of color processing up to the level of the double opponent cells in the blobs in V1 is understood in broad outline, a lot more work needs to be done on the physiology of the cells in V2 and V4. Responses of the double opponent cells in V1 correlate with observations of simultaneous color contrast, but probably not with object color constancy. Cells in V4 give responses very similar to human perception in displays that test object color constancy, but the variety of possible displays and the variety of cells to be tested is such that new findings are quite possible.

The existence of an area in macaque cortex (V4) that is particularly concerned with color has been correlated with a human condition called color agnosia. This is due to lesions at the junction of the inferomedial temporal and occipital lobes. People with this condition have a great deal of difficulty distinguishing one color from another, even though most other visual abilities are normal. The condition is frequently associated with prosopagnosia, which is the inability to recognize faces.

The final point that should be made is that, while color vision is treated as a separate heading in textbooks, and some areas in the visual system are more concerned with color than others, color is not processed in the visual system separately from form, shape, and movement. Cells in V1 outside the blobs, and also cells in V4, are specific for the orientation, size, and direction of movement of the stimulus, as well as its color. These areas are presumably involved in analyzing the total perception of a stimulus, with color being an important component, but not the only component of that perception.

Further reading

Daw NW (1968): Organisation for simultaneous color contrast. *Science* 158:942–944

Daw NW (1984): The psychology and physiology of colour vision. *Trend Neurosci* 7:330–335

Livingstone MS, Hubel DH (1984): Anatomy and physiology of a color system in the primate visual cortex. *J Neurosci* 4:309–356

Michael CR (1981): Columnar organisation of color cells in monkey striate cortex. *J Neurophysiol* 46:587–604

Pearlman AL, Birch J and Meadows JC (1979): Cerebral color blindness: an acquired defect in hue discrimination. *Ann Neurol* 5:253–261

Zeki SM (1983): Colour coding in the cerebral cortex: the reaction of cells in monkey visual cortex to wavelengths and colours. *Neuroscience* 9:741–765

Color Vision, Deficiencies

Leo M. Hurvich

The varieties of color vision deficiency are conventionally categorized as (1) anomalous trichromacy, (2) dichromacy, and (3) monochromacy. They are, respectively, three-variable, two-variable, and one-variable color vision systems, and their nature is best understood in the framework of a theoretical quantitative opponent-colors model that represents the way the normal three-variable color vision mechanism is organized. The normal trichromatic system is constituted of three independent color systems. Two are chromatic, red/green and yellow/blue, and one is achromatic, white/black.

In the opponent-colors model there are two linked processes or stages: (1) a photoreceptor level in the retina that is followed by (2) a neural one. At the cone photoreceptor stage, light is absorbed by three different photopigments, and chemical processes in them then trigger excitatory and inhibitory processes in the succeeding neural stages in the retina, lateral geniculate nucleus, and cortex. Figure 1a shows the three different photopigment absorption functions that have been measured for the normal eye using microspectrophotometric methods. These cone absorption spectra are arbitrarily labeled α, β, and γ.

Figure 1b shows the way the three opponent color responses of the normal eye—red/green, yellow/blue, and white/(black)—are distributed in the spectrum. Plus and minus directions represent opponency in each of the three paired opponent systems. These functions are based on the results of human psychophysical experiments. (The blackness response, which is measurable as a contrast phenomenon, is not shown in the figure. It is the mirror image of the whiteness curve.) Electrophysiological measures in nonhuman primates confirm the opponency concept at the cellular level and closely resemble the opponent-response sensitivities shown in the figure.

In the average normal human trichromatic eye, the cone photoreceptor responses and succeeding neural (perceptually correlated) events can be linked quantitatively in the following ways with exposure to spectral light of equal energy:

$$\text{red-green} = 0.37\,\alpha_\lambda + 1.66\,\gamma_\lambda - 2.23\,\beta_\lambda \tag{1}$$

$$\text{yellow-blue} = 0.06\,\beta_\lambda + 0.34\,\gamma_\lambda - 0.71\,\alpha_\lambda \tag{2}$$

$$\text{white-(black)} = 0.01\,\alpha_\lambda + 0.15\,\beta_\lambda + 0.85\,\gamma_\lambda \tag{3}$$

The α, β, and γ functions are the photoreceptor distribution functions, the numerical values are weighting terms, and the signed outcome in each equation provides the color code. Thus red and yellow and white are positive and green and blue negative. (The signs of the coded responses could be reversed with no change in concept.) For the average observer, perceived hue and its associated whiteness value for any spectral wavelength can be read directly from Figure 1b. Computed perceptual and discriminative indices based on these response curves are in excellent agreement with directly measured indices. Not only are the results of color mixture, wavelength, and saturation discrimination and the phenomena of color adaptation accounted for, but color deficiencies are also explainable in quantitative terms with this form of opponent-colors model.

Color vision abnormalities are either congenital and manifest genetic regularities or are acquired, i.e., develop during an individual's lifetime. The latter are usually caused by toxins, traumas (cerebral accidents), or hereditary and nonhereditary diseases. The incidence of congenital color deficiency is about 8% in male Caucasians and is appreciably lower among various Asiatic groups and such American groups as Indians, blacks, and Mexicans. The more common congenital defects (affecting the red/green system) are of a recessive mendelian type and are transmitted in a sex-linked fashion; grandchildren inherit these deficiencies from their grandfathers via daughters who

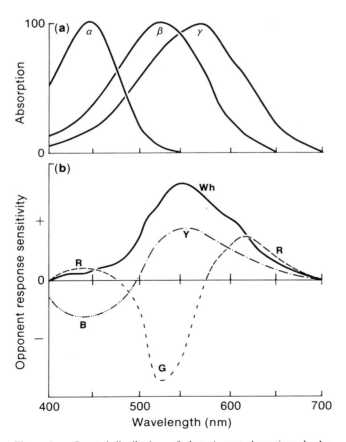

Figure 1. a. Spectral distributions of photopigment absorptions. b. Antagonistic or opponent red/green and yellow/blue response sensitivities, and achromatic whiteness response. The mirror image blackness curve is not shown.

are color-normal. Other defects have been attributed to incompletely dominant autosomal genes. The incidence of congenital deficiencies is some 20 times higher in males than in females, and of the various types of color deficiency, anomalous trichromacy accounts for somewhat more than half the deficiencies.

Like normal color vision, anomalous trichromacy is trichromatic but deviates from the normal system in several specific ways. If one or more of the α, β, and γ absorption functions of Figure 1a are distorted in form or if their spectral peak locations are shifted toward the short or long wave directions compared with those of the normal individual, these changes, assuming that the relations expressed in equations (1), (2), and (3) hold, will modify the forms and displace the spectral loci of the neural response curves of Figure 1b. Some individuals with such dislocated functions can discriminate colors with high precision along the three dimensions of normal color vision, namely, red/green, yellow/blue, and white/black but show imbalances in the way they perceive colors. The degree of imbalance will vary with the degree of spectral displacement of the photopigment distribution functions, and this expresses itself not only in the perceptual domain but also in the use of disproportionate amounts of stimulus primaries in making color matches as compared to normals. In making the following color match, for example,

$$v\,(535\ \text{nm}) + w\,(670\ \text{nm}) \equiv q(589\ \text{nm}) \qquad (4)$$

individuals with photopigment(s) assumed to be shifted toward shorter wavelengths require relatively more energy at 670 nm than at 535 nm. They are called *protanomalous*. Those with photopigment displacement(s) toward the longwave direction employ relatively greater amounts of the 535-nm stimulus to make this color match. They are called *deuteranomalous*.

In addition to spectral shifts in the photopigment functions and associated changes in the neural response functions, the latter are expressed with different degrees of efficiency in a population of anomalous observers. The red/green curve may, for example, vary from 100% efficiency to say, 10% or 3%. The variations in responsiveness are independent of the varieties of spectral displacements, and individuals with decremented red/green response systems may appropriately be labeled "color weak." This may occur even in the absence of a photopigment shift, and it has been suggested that such individuals be called neuteranomalous. Thus anomalous observers whose systems have two modes of possible variation, i.e., spectral shifts and variations in neural responsiveness, can run the gamut from those whose color matching behavior approximates a normal person's, but whose discriminative capacities are low, to those whose color matches may differ considerably from the normal but who are nonetheless extremely sharp color discriminators.

The yellow/blue chromatic system must also be considered in evaluating anomalous color vision, and rare cases of so-called tritanomaly are reported in the literature.

If the red/green chromatic function is reduced to zero efficiency level, i.e., it is lacking altogether or completely nonfunctioning, we have a dichromatic, two-variable system made up of only the yellow/blue and white/black response functions. Such individuals see only yellows and blues of varied saturations, and whites, grays, and blacks. Dichromats of this type

are colloquially termed red-green blind, and there are two subcategories. Deuteranopes have a whiteness function located at the spectral position shown in Figure 1b. Protanopes, like the protonomalous whose photopigment absorption functions are displaced toward short wavelengths, show displaced yellow/blue and achromatic response curves. A third form of dichromacy, called tritanopia, is extremely rare. It involves loss of the yellow/blue responses leaving only the red/green and whiteness responses. The chromatic response losses can occur because of central factors or, what is more widely believed for congenital defects, can result from the loss of one of the absorbing photopigment types; α in tritanopia, β in deuteranopia, γ in protanopia.

By simple extension, if both red/green and yellow/blue response mechanisms are lacking simultaneously, we have what is commonly called total color blindness or monochromatic color vision. Individuals of this type with good foveal vision and normal acuity see a world of objects differentiated only by lightness. They see only whites, grays, and blacks. A different form of monochromacy is also known in which there seems to be a lack of all cone function. It is called rod monochromacy or typical achromacy. In these cases, low visual acuity, central blind spots, nystagmus, and photophobia are commonly found. These individuals have poor vision in daylight but like the first type, the cone monochromats, they also see only whites, grays, and blacks and discriminate no hues whatsoever.

Color deficiencies are diagnosed by color matches, increment thresholds, measures of wavelength and saturation discrimination, and by locating the spectral wavelengths (if any) that appear neutral (achromatic). Such measurements are usually restricted to the laboratory. The most commonly used diagnostic tests are based on the pseudoisochromatic principle. These tests evaluate an individual's capacity to discriminate letters, geometric figures, or numerals of specified chromaticities from backgrounds of different chromaticities (e.g., the Ishihara plates). A different type of test is one that depends on an observer's ability to arrange a series of test colors in order of similarity (e.g., the Farnsworth-Munsell panel D-15 test). As a rule, a battery of tests of different kinds is used.

No treatment, whether drugs, vitamins, or exercises, has any demonstrable effect in improving deficiencies in *color vision*. Selective filter devices can cue a color-deficient person to the presence of a color difference by revealing a brightness difference to which he is sensitive, but such devices never bring with them the full experiential color world of the individual endowed with normal color vision.

Further reading

Fletcher R, Voke J (1985): *Defective Colour Vision*. Bristol: Adam Hilger

Hurvich LM (1972): Color vision deficiencies. In: *Handbook of Sensory Physiology*, vol 7/4, *Visual Psychophysics*. Jameson D, Hurvich LM, eds. Berlin: Springer-Verlag

Hurvich LM (1972): *Color Vision*. Sunderland, Mass: Sinauer

Jameson D (1972): Theoretical issues of color vision. In: *Handbook of Sensory Physiology*, vol 7/4, *Visual Psychophysics*. Jameson D, Hurvich LM, eds. Berlin: Springer-Verlag

Pokorny J, Smith VC, Verriest G, Pinckers, AJLG, eds (1979): *Congenital and Acquired Color Vision Defects*. New York: Grune & Stratton

Color Vision and Retinex Theory

Edwin H. Land

It is a cultural commonplace deriving from Newton that the color of an object in the world around us depends on the relative amounts of red, green, and blue light coming from the object to our eyes. In contradiction, it has long been known that the color of an object when it is part of a general scene will not change markedly with those considerable changes in the relative amounts of red, green, and blue light that characterize illumination from sunlight versus blue skylight versus gray daylight versus tungsten light versus fluorescent light. This contradiction is called *color constancy*. We need not examine the explanations of color constancy by Helmholtz and those who have followed him during the last century because, as the following experiments show, the paradox does not really exist: The color of an object is not determined by the composition of the light coming from the object.

The first group of experiments is carried out with an arrangement of real fruits and vegetables. A black and white photograph of the scene is shown in Figure 1. In a dark room with black walls, three illuminating projectors with clear slides in the slide holders are directed on the scene. The brightness of the projectors is individually controllable. An interference filter passing 450 nm is placed in front of one projector, 550 nm in front of the second, and 610 nm in front of the third. The measurements in this experiment are all carried out with a telescopic photometer that reads the flux toward the eye from a circular area about 8 mm in diameter on the surface of an object. The readings are in watts per steradian per square meter. All readings are made with light from only one projector at a time. Three synchronized camera shutters on the illuminating projectors make possible comparison of the colors in the fruit and vegetables as seen with continuous illumination and as seen with illumination for only a fraction of a second.

The meter is directed at an orange, the fluxes toward the eye on the three wavebands are set equal to each other, and the orange is observed when the whole scene is illuminated with the combined light from the three illuminators. The orange is orange-colored. The process is repeated for a green pepper so that the identical radiation comes to the eye—the same three equal wattages as came from the orange. The green pepper is green. Similarly, when the identical radiation reaches the eye from a yellow banana, the banana is yellow. When the identical radiation reaches the eye from a dark red pepper, the pepper is dark and the pepper is red.

Observations in a pulse of light

One of the most important experiments in this group is to compare the scene as viewed in continuous illumination with the scene viewed in a fractional second pulse. In view of the historic tendency to involve adaptation and eye motion as causal factors in color constancy, it is gratifying to see that for every new setting, as we turn our attention from object to object, the colors seen in a pulse are correct.

Whether the scene is viewed in a fractional second pulse or in continuous illumination, straw is straw-color, rye bread is rye-bread-color, limes are lime-color, green apples are green and red apples are red, with the illuminators of the scene so set in each case that the very same ratio of wattages of long-, middle-, and short-wave radiation comes to the eye from each of the objects in this list. That is, observed through a spectrophotometer, they would all look alike. Since this experiment establishes that the color of an object is not a function of the composition of the light coming from the object, there is nothing surprising about the failure of the objects to change color when the composition of the illumination changes: color constancy is the name of a nonexistent paradox.

Color and wavelength composition

In Figure 1 a pile of pigment is located in front of the peppers. The pigment is red lead oxide, or minium, referred to in Newton's *Opticks* (1704) in Proposition X, Problem V. "Minium reflects the least refrangible or red-making rays most copiously, and thence appears red. . . . Every Body reflects the Rays of its own Colour more copiously than the rest, *and from their excess and predominance in the reflected Light has its Colour.*" The demonstrations in this group of experiments prove that the part of Newton's proposition that we have italicized is incorrect. When the scene is so illuminated that the minium sends to the eye fluxes with the same three equal wattages, the minium continues to look its own brilliant orange-red color—even though there is not at all an "excess and predominance in the reflected light" of "red-making

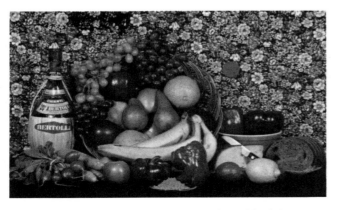

Figure 1. Arrangement of real fruits and vegetables with minium.

rays." This group of experiments leads to the first statement in Retinex theory:

1. The composition of the light from an area in an image does not specify the color of that area.

Lightness

When the fruit and vegetable scene is illuminated by light of one waveband, we observe that the very light objects stay very light and the very dark objects stay very dark as we alter the brightness of the illumination over nearly the whole range between extinction and maximum illumination. For example, with middle-wave illumination the red pepper will be always almost black and the green pepper always a light gray green. This situation will be reversed when we change to long wave illumination; that is, the red pepper will always be light and the green pepper always dark.

Based on these observations, it is reasonable to hypothesize that an object which always looks light with middle wave illumination on the scene and always looks dark with long wave illumination on the scene will look green when the scene is illuminated with both illuminators and will continue to look green as we change the relative brightness of the long and middle wave illuminators and hence the relative fluxes from the object to the eye. Similarly, an object which is dark in middle-wave illumination and light in long-wave illumination will look red when the scene is illuminated with both illuminators and will continue to look red as we change the relative brightnesses of the two illuminators. Similar relationships can be established for short-wave illumination.

The retinex computation

If color can indeed be predicted on the basis of the three lightnesses at a point, we are led to the question of how to predict for each waveband separately, each of the three lightnesses of a point in an image. We would like to know how to compute the number on which lightness is based in the hope that we will find that a given trio of numbers will always be a single color, a color uniquely corresponding to the given trio. We will call each member of this trio a "designator," the computed numerical measure on one waveband of the lightness of an area seen as part of the whole field of view.

A new and relatively simple technique for this computation of the designator is proposed here. Previous Retinex techniques involve some kind of comparison between the flux (on one waveband) coming to the eye from a point on the object and flux (on that same waveband) arriving from points in remote, as well as contiguous, areas. These comparisons involve edges, gradients, thresholds, and pathways; they provide the average of the relationships between a given point and a large number of other points in the field of view. In all Retinex theory, the criteria are that the value determined be independent of uniformity and intensity of illumination and be achievable with an exposure less than a millisecond, i.e., independent of adaptation. The new technique, instead of utilizing an average of the relationships between the flux from the point of interest and the flux from each of many other points in the field, utilizes the ratio of the flux from the point of interest to an average, weighted in an unusual way, of all the fluxes from all the points in the field. The designator is the logarithm of this ratio.

It is easily shown that this average must not be a simple average taken over the whole field of view. Figure 2a shows a collage of black, white, and gray areas, randomly distributed and randomly surrounded. If area 1 reflects 8% of the light

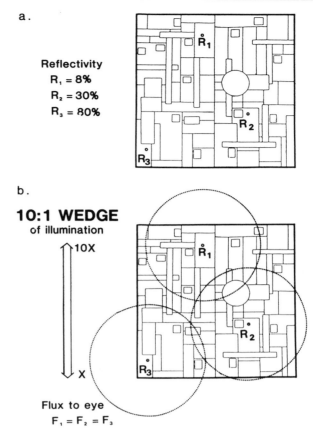

a.

Reflectivity
$R_1 = 8\%$
$R_2 = 30\%$
$R_3 = 80\%$

b.

10:1 WEDGE
of illumination

10X

X

Flux to eye
$F_1 = F_2 = F_3$

Figure 2. A collage of black, white, and gray matte papers is shown in a and b. R_1 reflects 8% of the light falling on it, R_2, 30%, and R_3, 80%. In b when the illumination is so adjusted by neutral wedges in the illuminator that the flux to the eye (F_1) from R_1 equals the flux to the eye (F_2) from R_2 equals the flux to the eye (F_3) from R_3, the observer will notice that the black stays black, the gray stays gray, and the white stays white even though the three measured fluxes to the eye are identical. The dotted circle in b represents a 16-degree diameter field.

falling on it, area 2, 30%, and area 3, 80%, the first will look dark, almost black, the second, a middle gray, and the third, almost white. If the illumination is so adjusted by neutral wedges in the illuminator (as in Fig. 2b) that the flux to the eye from R_1 equals the flux to the eye from R_2, equals the flux to the eye from R_3, the observer will scarcely notice. The nearly black area stays dark, the middle gray area stays gray, and the white area stays white—even though the three measured fluxes to the eye are identical. If we now take the ratio of the flux from R_1 to the average flux for the whole field, and the ratio of the flux from R_2 to the average flux for the whole field, and the ratio of the flux from R_3 to the average flux for the whole field, these three ratios will equal each other. Therefore they do not provide numbers correlated with the fact that R_1 looks almost black, and R_2 looks gray, and R_3 looks white. Clearly, the overall average cannot be used for the denominator in the relationship we seek.

If, instead of the overall average, we were to use the average flux from the contiguous areas (to give the value of the denominator) we would have to be concerned about the randomness of this kind of average because of the arbitrary reflectivities, and the smallness of the population, of contiguous areas.

A search for an operative compromise between an average

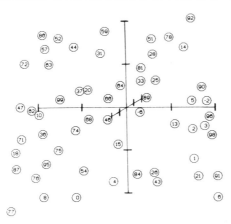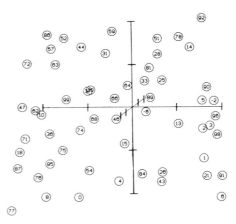

Figure 3. Stereoscopic view of Retinex 3-space: left-eye view on the left. A stereoscopic colored version of the 3-space appears in Land (*Proc Nat Acad Sci* 1986). Here we are limited to black and white. The numbers refer to the Coloraid papers (Table 1) which made up several Mondrians. Three designators for each of those papers were determined according to the computation described here, and the colored papers were located in the color 3-space. In this diagram, numbers that run along a diagonal from the lower left to the upper right, 77 (black), 76, 75, 74, 68, 66, 64, 81, 78, and 92 (white) refer to papers that lie on the gray line running from black through gray to white; other color domains are the following:

blues, 52, 72, and 86; dark browns, 8 and 0; browns, 43 and 84; greens, 18, 36, 37, 46, 62, and 71; blue greens, 44, 47, and 63; orange, 21; purples, 14, 20, 28, 33, 51, and 89; reds, 6, 91, 96, and 98; yellows, 1, 3, and 5. Note that the reds in the Mondrian are numbered 6, 91, 96, and 98. The algorithm leads to designators for these areas that are close enough in value to place them in one domain in the 3-space in spite of the fact that in the Mondrian each of these red areas was surrounded by a different variety of colored areas and in spite of the fact that the illumination of each red area in the Mondrian could be different in composition from that of the other red areas.

taken over the whole field and an average taken over the contiguous areas gives promising results. For example, if, for the numerator, we use the flux per unit area over a 4-arc-minute field, and for the denominator, the flux per unit area averaged over a 16-degree field (Fig. 2b), the ratios correlate with the

appearance of the black, the gray, and the white areas, and the logarithms of these ratios give a trio of numbers which plot in the Retinex color three-space (Fig. 3) at the correct locations for black, gray, and white. Even in this simple form, this measuring technique will satisfactorily locate a point in

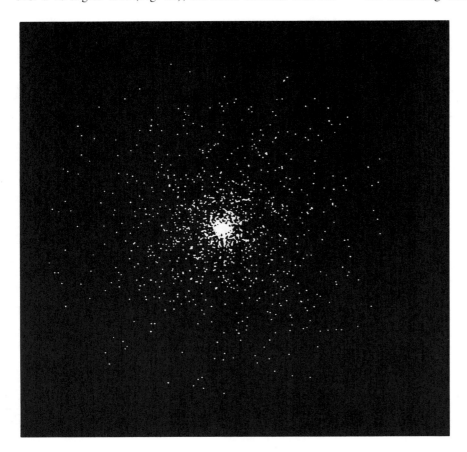

Figure 4. The pattern of sensitivity for the photometer reading of the denominator. The angle from the center to the outer dots (5.4 cm in this figure) is 12 degrees. One half the dots are inside a circle of radius 2 degrees. (The corresponding radius of the numerator is 2 arc-minutes.) The density of dots, which was chosen empirically, here varies approximately as the inverse square of the radius.

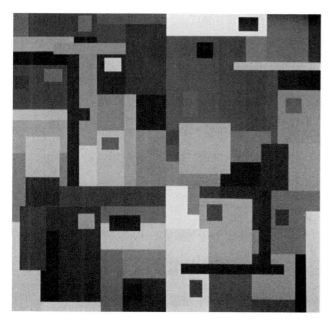

Figure 5. Black and white photograph of color Mondrian.

the color space in agreement with the three designators for each area in a colored Mondrian, and for the areas in the Macbeth color cards, for arrangements of fruits and vegetables and flowers, for clothing and real scenes.

Experiments, however, have shown that the flux from the extremes of the field of vision is somehow a significant contributor to the average. For example, with very large projected images, the radiation can be excluded from reaching the screen in an annular domain around the object of interest. Even though the radius of the outer circumference of the annulus may be relatively large, the average of the radiation beyond the annulus will for each of the three wavebands give a useful denominator; that is, it will produce a designator that meets our criteria of mapping lightnesses of equal value together in the color space.

Is there a pattern of sensitivity that would satisfy the condi-

tions of the experiments we have described so far? A pattern that seems promising is one which, although suggested by the decreasing concentration of retinal cones with increasing radius, was actually arrived at empirically (Fig. 4). We have designed this pattern into the photometer so that the small angle reading for the numerator is taken through the center of it, and the wide angle reading for the denominator utilizes the whole pattern which now covers more than twice the area of the circle in Figure 2b. This technique for computation of the designator in Retinex theory has the appeal of intuitive simplicity and carries out all the tasks implicit in color constancy. Furthermore, it has the competence not possessed by earlier algorithms for generating Mach bands. These observations lead to the second statement in Retinex theory:

2. The color of a unit area is determined by a trio of numbers each computed on a single waveband to give the relationship for that waveband between the flux from a unit area and the specially weighted average of the fluxes from the rest of the scene.

When an image of a colored Mondrian (Fig. 5 and Table 1), a collage of colored rectangles, is formed and the computational technique proposed is pursued, it is found that the 3-space is populated in an orderly way. The points on one of the internal diagonals turn out to look black at one end, run through gray, and are white at the other end of the diagonal. There is a domain in which the greens reside, another for the reds, still another for the blues, and yet another for the yellows. It is a triumph of this computational technique that the overall variation in the composition of the illumination in terms of flux at a given wavelength or in terms of relative flux between wavelengths does not disturb the reliability with which a paper that looks red, no matter where it resides in the Mondrian, will have the same three designators, as the other papers that look red. It will therefore be part of a family of reds which appears in one domain of the 3-space. Similarly, all the blues or greens or yellows, wherever resident in the Mondrian and however haply illuminated, will appear in their appropriate domains in the 3-space (Fig. 3). It is the computation that leads each paper to have its position in the 3-space; the proof of the pudding is that all things that appear in the same region of the 3-space are the same color as one another,

Table 1. Coloraid Papers

Location #	Coloraid	Location #	Coloraid	Location #	Coloraid
1	Y T1	36	YG T1	75	gray 7A
2	Y T3	37	GYG T4	76	gray 8
3	R T1	43	O S1	77	black
4	Y S3	44	GBG T4	78	gray 1A
5	Y T4	46	YGY T4	81	gray 2
6	RO hue	47	BV hue	84	sienna brown
8	RO S3	51	V T4	86	cobalt blue
10	VBV hue	52	B T1	87	navy blue
13	RVR hue	54	YO S3	89	magenta
14	RV T3	57	BG T1	90	rose red
15	YOY S1	59	BVB T4	91	life red
18	G hue	62	BG S2	92	white
20	V hue	63	GBG T2	95	YG S3
21	YOY hue	64	gray 4A	96	RO T3
25	ROR S3	66	gray 5A	98	ROR T1
26	Y S1	68	gray 6A	99	GYG S2
28	VRV T2	71	GBG hue	0	RO S2
31	VBV T2	72	BVB hue	−2	RO T4
33	RV S1	74	gray 7	−6	ORO S1

Note: These numbered Coloraid papers were among those used to make up Mondrians such as the one shown in Figure 5. The designators of the papers were measured and the papers were located in the color space (Fig. 3).

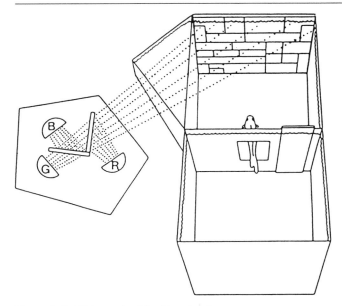

Figure 6. Goldfish entering Mondrian chamber.

whatever their history in terms of geography and illumination on the Mondrian may have been. Thus we arrive at the third statement in Retinex theory:

3. The trio of numbers as computed by the Retinex ratiometer designates a point in Retinex 3-space which is the color of the unit area.

Applications of retinex theory and the retinex computation

The predictive power of the computation is shown not merely by these examples but also by many other experiments. Of fundamental importance is the ability of the computation to predict darks, lights, shadows, highlights, light sources, and extended areas in surrounds with extremely low reflectivity. As a quite different example, the color of an area located on the Mondrian can be predicted and determined, while the flux to the eye is held constant, by modifying the designators within the area by computed changes in the rest of the field, for each waveband separately. Thus, the area can be changed from a specified white to a specified dark purple—without changing the flux to the eye from the area—by changes in the whole Mondrian computed for each waveband. In an important corollary experiment the area which is being changed from white to purple is surrounded by a very wide black border (produced by blocking the light at the slide holder of the illuminating projector). The computed changes in the Mondrian, which have altered the designators for the area to make it white or purple, continue to be effective in the presence of the wide black border. This technique was employed as a tool, using an observer with a split brain, to show that the Retinex computation, wherever in the retinal-cortical system it is carried out, is long range and involves cortical participation.

A most dramatic application of Retinex theory is the quantitative prediction of the colors available in the classical experiment of projecting with red and white light. (Two black and white pictures, one being the long-wave color separation image and the other being the middle-wave separation image, are projected in superposition with red and neutral filters to give a remarkable gamut of appropriate colors.) If the two projections of the red and white light are made in combination through a large long-wave transmitting filter and then through a large middle-wave transmitting filter and then through a large short-wave transmitting filter, the ratiometer, reading the image on each of the three wavebands separately, will predict the three designators for locating the colors in the 3-space.

D. Ingle undertook the investigation of the question: "Is the goldfish a Retinex animal?" The answer is dramatically in the affirmative: a goldfish selects a color he has been trained for when he is removed from the training tank and placed in a tank at one end of which is a Mondrian. In a series of tests, the Mondrian is so illuminated as to send to the fish's eye from an area of the color he is trained for the same number of photons of the same frequency as came from each of many other colors in the Mondrian under some standard illumination (Fig. 6).

N. Daw's early discovery of double-opponent cells in the goldfish opened the way for correlation between the opponent ideas of Hering and physiological investigations. This brief article will not examine the coordinate transformations that take Retinex theory into the domain of double-opponent cells in the visual pathway.

M. Livingstone and D. Hubel's 1984 results "suggest that a system involved in the processing of color information, especially color-spatial interactions, runs parallel to and separate from the orientation-specific system. Color, encoded in three coordinates by the major blob cell types, red-green, yellow-blue, and black-white, can be transformed into the three coordinates, red, green, and blue, of the Retinex algorithm of Land."

S. Zeki has discovered color-reading cells in the V4 region of the prestriate visual cortex of the rhesus monkey. The image of a Mondrian is formed on the retina of the anesthetized monkey, and Mondrian experiments analogous to those carried out on humans are carried out with the animal. The results for the monkey, as reported by his cortical cells, are strikingly similar to the results for humans.

Further reading

Early papers on retinex theory
Land E (1959): Color vision and the natural image, Parts I and II. *Proc Nat Acad Sci* 45:115–129 and 636–644.
Land E, McCann J (1971): Lightness and Retinex theory. *J Opt Soc Am* 61:1–11
McCann J, McKee S, Taylor T (1976): Quantitative studies in Retinex Theory. *Vis Res* 16:445–458

Recent papers on retinex theory
Land E (1983): Recent advances in Retinex theory and some implications for cortical computations: Color vision and the natural image. *Proc Nat Acad Sci* 80:5163–5169
Land E, Hubel D, Livingstone M, Perry S, Burns M (1983): Color-generating interactions across the corpus callosum. *Nature* 303:616–618
Land E (1986): Recent advances in Retinex theory. *Vision Res* 26(1):7–21
Land E (1986): An alternative technique for the computation of the designator in the Retinex Theory of color vision. *Proc Nat Acad Sci* 83:3078–3080

Related papers in neurophysiology
Livingstone M, Hubel D (1984): Anatomy and physiology of a color system in the primate visual cortex. *J Neurosci* 4:309–356
Zeki S (1980): The representation of colours in the cerebral cortex. *Nature* 284:412–418

Cone Photoreceptors, Color Specificities

Teruya Ohtsuka

Cone photoreceptors (cones) in the vertebrate retina mediate color vision. Cones are composed of four parts; an outer segment, an inner segment, a cell body, and a synaptic terminal (pedicle) (Fig. 1). The outer segment is made of numerous infoldings of the plasma membrane, which contains a photosensitive substance (visual pigment). Microspectrophotometric studies have shown that individual cones contain one of the three different visual pigments whose absorbances are maximal for red, green, and blue lights. Three sets of visual pigments are commonly found in vertebrates; for example, the absorbance maxima lie at 625, 530, and 455 nm in the goldfish; 623, 522, and 462 nm in the turtle; 567, 514, and 461 in the pigeon; 567, 535, and 415 in the monkey (*Macaca*); and 558, 531, and 419 nm in the human. These varieties of absorbance maxima are probably related to the adaptation to the light environment of the habitats.

When illuminated, the voltage across cone membrane hyperpolarizes; action potentials are not generated. Hyperpolarization of cones follows with breakdown of visual pigments, which depends on the intensity as well as on the wavelength of incident light. In the dark, a cyclic nucleotide, cyclic guanosine monophosphate (cGMP), maintains a high permeability to Na^+ in the outer segment membrane, and thus extracellular Na^+ flows inward according to its electrochemical gradient. Bleaching of the visual pigment by light activates an enzyme phosphodiesterase which hydrolyzes cGMP. Reduction of cytoplasmic cGMP lowers membrane permeability to Na^+. Since permeability to other ions (primarily K^+) are insensitive to light, the decrease of Na^+ influx results in membrane hyperpolarization. In this way, the energy of incident light is transformed to changes of membrane potential; this, in turn, regulates neurotransmitter release from the synaptic terminal that conveys the visual signal to second-order neurons and beyond.

Intracellular recordings from many vertebrate cones have revealed that the membrane potential in the dark is -10 to -30 mV and the hyperpolarizing amplitude to very bright lights saturates at about 20 mV. The relation between the response amplitude and the logarithmic scale of applied light intensity follows a sigmoidal curve covering an intensity range of 10^3. A single photon evokes a responses of about 10 μV in amplitude, the value almost 100 times smaller than that of rod photoreceptors.

Spectral sensitivity of cones is determined by measuring response amplitudes to monochromatic lights (380–760 nm); the sensitivity at each wavelength is defined by a reciprocal of the light intensity that produces a threshold amplitude. Since intracellular recording from cones in the primate retina is extremely difficult due to their small size (about 2 μm in diameter), the light-evoked current through the outer segment is used instead of membrane potential changes. In many vertebrate retinas, three sets of cones with different spectral sensitivities were found; for example, maximal sensitivities are at 611,

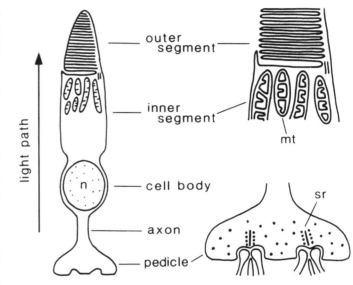

Figure 1. Schematic illustration of the cone photoreceptor. The outer segment is made of numerous infoldings of the plasma membrane which contains the visual pigment. The inner segment is packed with mitochondria (mt), and the cell body contains a nucleus (n). The axon terminates in the synaptic ending, pedicle, containing several *synaptic ribbons* (sr). Dendrites of second-order neurons, bipolar cells, and horizontal cells, invaginate into several pits in the basal surface of pedicle and form the triad of postsynaptic elements. Note the light-sensitive outer segment situates at the opposite end of incident light.

529, and 462 nm in the carp; at 630, 550, and 460 nm in the turtle; and at 570 and 540 nm in monkey (*Macaca*) cones (no blue-sensitive cone has yet been studied). These cones with sensitivity peaks at red, green, and blue spectra are referred to as red-sensitive, green-sensitive, and blue-sensitive cones. Each of the spectral sensitivity curves coincides with the absorption spectrum of the corresponding visual pigment. Thus the first stage of color vision in vertebrates is initiated by the trichromatic types of cones, as proposed by Thomas Young.

In some vertebrate cones, spectral sensitivity curves do not match the absorption spectra of corresponding visual pigments. This difference is due to the filtering effect of the intraocular media (lens and cornea) and retinal cells. An extreme example is found in the reptilian and avian cones containing oil droplets, small lipid balls made of various colored carotinoids located in the distal inner segments. Since the shorter wavelength of incident light is absorbed by the oil droplets prior to reaching the outer segment, the sensitivity peak shifts to a longer wavelength from the absorbance maximum of visual pigments. In turtle green-sensitive cone, for example, maximal sensitivity is shifted by about 30 nm from the maximal absorbance (522 nm) of the green-absorbing pigment.

The relation between spectral sensitivity of cones and the color of oil droplets provides a reliable morphological basis for identification of three chromatic types of cones. It is useful for the study of neuronal networks underlying color information processing in vertebrate retina.

Cones are not functionally independent but interact with neighboring cones and second-order neurons. For example, cones are coupled to their neighbors at fine processes emanating from the pedicle. The membrane potential of cones is also affected by the activity of horizontal cells. The signals sent from cones to horizontal cells come back again to cones through sign-inverting synapses. This negative feedback signal is thought to evoke a depolarization in a horizontal cell which shows opponent spectral responses.

Further reading

Davson H (1980): *Physiology of the Eye*. London: Churchill Livingston

Fuortes MGF, ed (1972): *Physiology of Photoreceptor Organs. Handbook of Sensory Physiology VII/2*. Berlin: Springer

Nunn BJ, Schnapf JL, Baylor DA (1984): Spectral sensitivity of single cones in the retina of *Macaca fascicularis*. *Nature* 309:264–266

Ohtsuka T (1985): Relation of spectral types to oil droplets in cones of turtle retina. *Science* 229:874–877

Electroretinogram, Electroretinography

John C. Armington

The electroretinogram (ERG) is a compound potential produced by the layers of the retina in response to visual stimulation. Electroretinography pertains to the study and recording of this potential. The ERG is important because of its value in basic physiological research, in monitoring peripheral action during the course of psychophysical investigation, and in the diagnosis of a variety of visual disorders. The first ERGs were recorded well over a century ago, and there has been continuing study of their properties ever since. The ERG is better understood than most mass action potentials, and particularly those that can be recorded with electrodes that are some distance from the source.

The electroretinogram appears between electrodes placed on opposite sides of the retina in response to a change in the incident light, but it may also be obtained with electrodes that are placed more remotely as, for example, on the cornea and the back of the eye. The ERG is conveniently recorded from the human eye with an electrode supported in a contact lens and worn by the subject. The signal that is collected is recorded with conventional electrophysiological instrumentation.

Two types of stimulation may be used to elicit the electroretinogram. With the first, the eye is presented with a simple flash to produce transient stimulation of the retina; with the second, the eye is presented with an alternating pattern of bright and dark stripes or checkers whose luminances are exchanged periodically. The effects produced by the two methods are not the same. A flash produces a brief increment in the illumination of broad retinal regions through the action of stray light that is scattered or reflected from the primary image area. An alternating pattern, on the other hand, produces a small local response because the stray light beyond the image area is steady and, thus, ineffective as a stimulus.

The electroretinogram has a multiphasic waveform that is shaped from the contributions of several underlying activities, any of which may be more or less prominent. The stimulus characteristics, the state of the eye's adaptation, the species of the subject, and the recording conditions will all affect the result. Examples of ERGs, illustrating the principal features, are shown in Figure 1.

The names that have been given to the various peaks are identified in the figure. The a-, b-, and c-waves are fundamental to any discussion of the ERG. They are superimposed upon a more or less steady resting potential. The d-wave may appear when the stimulus is shut off. Several approaches have been used to sort out the components of the ERG, including the anatomical-physiological, the photopic-scotopic, and the flash versus patterned stimulus approach.

The first approach has succeeded in identifying the cells and the mechanisms that produce certain peaks and components, particularly those that occur in the early parts of the response. Current knowledge supports the assignments of com-

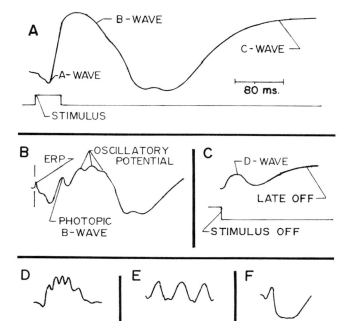

Figure 1. Representative ERG waveforms. Actual amplitudes and latencies vary widely. An upward deflection indicates positivity of the front of the retina with respect to the back. A. Typical of the scotopic response of the dark-adapted eye to a bright flash. B. This panel shows the relative timing of several waves; the early receptor potential (ERP) is not seen in actual recordings with the other components because it appears at higher stimulus levels. Oscillatory potentials are superimposed on the scotopic b-wave. C. The d-wave or off-effect appears when the stimulus is terminated. It may be followed by a succession of slow waves. D. The ERG of the predominantly photopic eye of the turtle has prominent oscillatory potentials. E. Photopic responses to a flickering stimulus. F. The response to an alternating pattern.

ponent to structure that follow, but undoubtedly future research will result in more complete knowledge and perhaps some revision. The earliest component arises with virtually no latency from photo pigment isomerization in the distal parts of the receptors and hence is called the early receptor potential (ERP). This component is small and thus is recorded only with very intense stimuli. It is followed by the a-wave whose initial limb arises from the proximal parts of the receptors. There is some evidence that the prominent features of the b-wave are produced by Mueller cells throughout the retina. They produce their signal in response to potassium ions that are released primarily in the inner and outer plexiform retinal

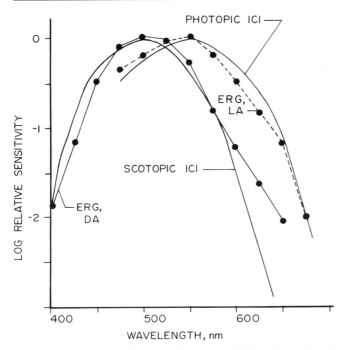

Figure 2. Spectral sensitivity of the light-adapted (LA) and dark-adapted (DA) ERG compared with the psychophysical photopic and scotopic ICI functions.

layers as a result of visual action. The peaks of the oscillatory potential have been localized to different depths within the bipolar layer. The c-wave has been shown to arise within the pigment epithelium cells at the back of the retina.

The photopic-scotopic approach attempts to separate components that are a consequence of stimulation of the rod or of the cone systems of the retina. Separation may be achieved by adapting the eye to appropriate light levels, using narrow wavelength band stimuli that favor one or the other mechanism, selecting subjects who have an impairment of one or the other system, or in other ways. Responses generated under scotopic and photopic conditions may both show a- and b-waves. The success in isolating scotopic and photopic components is judged by how well the spectral sensitivities of the electrical responses match corresponding psychophysical curves (Fig. 2). The terms photopic and scotopic a- and b-waves are sometimes used when these waves can be discerned in the response recordings.

The two kinds of stimulation in general use form the basis for the third analytical approach. Flash responses are elicited by stimuli that produce transient increases in overall retinal illumination. Pattern responses are produced by stimuli whose structure periodically undergoes temporal change. For example, a checkerboard is frequently used as a pattern for alternation. Responses are elicited by periodically interchanging the elements; that is, black checks abruptly become white, and white become black. It has been claimed that responses to pattern differ fundamentally from those to flashes because they give evidence of lateral interaction effects in the retina.

Information gathered with one approach may bear on that gathered with another. Most physiological work, where the attempt is made to assign components of the ERG to retinal structures, is based upon experiments with stimulus flashes.

If ERGs are elicited by individual flashes or by slow flicker in the human, they will tend to be dominated by scotopic features. More rapid flicker (above 20 Hz) will result in photopic activity. The responses produced by alternating patterns are predominantly photopic unless the patterns are very dim.

Applications of electroretinography

The electroretinogram has found widespread use in assessing visual function. Three areas of application are considered here: psychophysics, comparative study of vision, and clinical diagnosis of visual disorders.

Much current knowledge of visual function is based on psychophysical rather than direct physiological investigation. The ERG, which can be recorded from the same subjects that are used for psychophysics, makes it possible to coordinate the two types of investigation. The ERG has contributed significantly to the current knowledge of spectral sensitivity, light and dark adaptation, and color vision. It is useful in studying the peripheral areas of the visual field that are often difficult to work with psychophysically. Figure 2 compares the spectral sensitivities of the human ERG and of psychophysical thresholds (ICI luminosity curves) under photopic and scotopic conditions. Agreement, but not identity, is apparent. The spectral sensitivity of the dark-adapted eye also compares well with that of the rod pigment, rhodopsin.

The eyes of different animals vary rather remarkably, being adapted through evolution for a variety of habitats and ways of living. These variations are reflected in the ERG. One striking difference is between nocturnal and diurnal retinas. The former emphasize scotopic and the latter photopic features. Work with the ERG has helped show that specialization is seldom complete. Although a retina may be specialized for day or night vision, it will generally retain some function at all levels.

The electroretinogram has found its widest application in the diagnosis of visual disorders. It is often recorded in the clinic together with the visually evoked cortical potential, a signal arising within the brain, and the electrooculogram, an indicator of the retinal resting potential. Most clinical work has been done with flash stimuli. With these it is possible to distinguish a number of cogenital conditions, such as various forms of color blindness, day blindness, and night blindness. A more serious disease is retinitis pigmentosa, which leads to total blindness. Its progressive forms can be detected very early by an increase in ERG latency. The response becomes severely reduced in amplitude or extinguished as the disease progresses. Growth in amplitude is seen in the flash ERG when it is used to follow visual development in normal infants; it is extremely small at birth but increases rapidly during the first months of life. Patterned stimuli are useful for evaluating local retinal areas. Much current research is directed toward assessing the value of such stimuli in evaluating the condition of the inner retinal layers.

Further reading

Armington JC (1974): *The Electroretinogram.* New York: Academic Press

Berson EL (1981): Electrical phenomena in the retina. In: *Adlers's Physiology of the Eye: Clinical Application,* 7th ed. Moses RA, ed. St. Louis: Mosby

Carr RE, Siegel IM (1982): *Visual Electrodiagnostic Testing.* Baltimore: Williams and Wilkins

Eye-Head Coordination

Emilio Bizzi

To direct head and eyes toward a target and ultimately fixate it with the fovea, an animal must solve three problems. First, he must compute the angular distance between his foveal lines of sight and the target to be acquired. This angular distance is referred to as retinal error; its absolute magnitude will determine the amplitude of the saccadic eye movement that will be produced. Second, the animal must initiate a head movement that will be compatible in amplitude with the saccadic eye movement. Third, since the eyes usually move first and with higher velocity than the head, their lines of sight will reach and fixate the target while the head is still moving. To stabilize his eyes with respect to a stationary target during head movement, the animal must perform a rotational eye movement that, by being opposite in direction from the movement of the head, but equal to it in amplitude and velocity, allows the fovea to remain constantly on the target. This movement is termed compensatory.

Since in vertebrates the head begins to move, on the average, 10–30 msec after the initiation of the saccade, relatively large saccades (more than 10–30 msec in duration) will continue to take place while the head is moving. A case in point is shown in Figure 1b, which illustrates coordinated eye and head movements made in response to a target at 30° eccentricity, together with the sum of these movements, the gaze. Figure 1a displays the record of a saccadic eye movement made by the same animal in response to the same target while its head was artificially restrained. A comparison of the saccade in (a) and the gaze in (b) shows that the target was acquired with the same precision in both instances. The decrease in saccadic amplitude during head movement reflects an adjustment of the central eye movement program induced by head movement. In vertebrates, vestibular impulses have been shown to be responsible for the decrease of saccadic eye move-

ments. The crucial role of these impulses in monkeys was demonstrated by surgically interrupting the pathway linking the vestibular receptors to the vestibular nuclei. The reflex mode of organization greatly simplifies the task of the systems required for programming eye-head coordination. The eye and head movements can be programmed independently, since the vestibular system automatically nullifies any displacements of the fovea from the target produced by head movement.

The role of feedback from peripheral sensory organs (vestibular and neck afferents) also includes the control and generation of movements that stabilize the eyes with respect to the target during head movement. This spatial stabilization is accomplished by a movement of the eyes opposite in direction from that of head but of equal amplitude and velocity, thereby compensating for the head movement. It has long been known that compensatory eye movements are critically influenced by signals from vestibular receptors and neck proprioceptors. In monkeys, Dichgans and colleagues have shown that ocular stabilization during active head movements is due mainly to the vestibulo-ocular reflex. However, other species and humans rely on both the vestibular system and the neck loop. Experimental evidence also indicates that ocular stabilization is completely adequate in the absence of visual control.

A different strategy of eye-head coordination is observed during smooth tracking of a slowly moving target. Humans, monkeys, and cats use a combination of eye and head movements to track a moving visual stimulus. During eye-head tracking, the gaze (the sum of eye and head movements) remains on target just as accurately when the head is free as when the head is fixed and only the eyes pursue the target. Although the gaze is on target with and without head movement, the eye movements differ greatly in the two cases. The primary effect of freeing the head is that smooth pursuit is

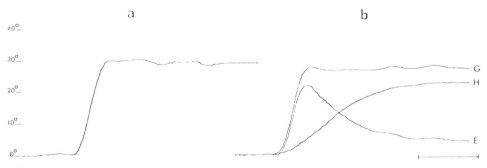

Figure 1. Comparison of eye saccades and gaze. a. Eye saccades, with head fixed, in response to a suddenly appearing target. b. Coordinated eye saccade (E) and head movement (H), with head free, in response to the same target. The gaze movement (G) represents the sum of E and H. Note the remarkable similarity of the eye saccade in (a) and the gaze trajectory in (b), as well as the reduced amplitude of the saccade in (b). Time calibration 100 msec. From Morasso et al (1973): *Exp Brain Res* 16:492–500, reprinted with permission.

accomplished almost entirely by the head movement system, while the eyes tend to remain fairly stationary in the center of the orbit.

Investigations of the mechanism for coordinating eye and head movements during the smooth pursuit of a slowly moving target revealed the presence, in the central nervous system (CNS), of a neural signal representing target velocity in space. There is evidence that this signal drives both the eye and the head movement centers. During normal smooth pursuit with the head free, the head follows this hypothesized command with a lag that depends on the activation time of the neck musculature. The eyes, however, appear to receive not only the postulated smooth pursuit signal, but also a signal generated by the activation of the vestibular system. This second signal specifies movements opposite in direction from the head movement and proportional to it. The combination of the two signals in some part of the oculomotor system results in an eye movement with an amplitude nearly equal to the difference between the amplitudes of the target and head movements. Since this difference is small, smooth pursuit with eyes and head consists mainly of head tracking.

In conclusion, there are interesting similarities and contrasts between the coordination of eye-head movement elicited by a stationary and by a moving target. The vestibular apparatus plays a crucial role in both strategies, and both strategies depend on a signal delivered in parallel and approximately simultaneously to eye and head motor systems. These similarities indicate that the two strategies have a common structural organization. But while in the visually triggered mode, eye and head movements depend critically on the retinal error signal, during smooth pursuit they depend on a central representation of target motion in space. These different commands for triggered and smooth pursuit are presumably produced by different calculations and may be produced in different regions of the CNS.

Further reading

Dichgans J, Bizzi E, Morasso P, Tagliasco V (1974): The role of vestibular and neck afferents during eye-head coordination in the monkey. *Brain Res* 71:225–232

Lanman J, Bizzi E, Allum J (1978): The coordination of eye and head movement during smooth pursuit. *Brain Res* 153:39–53

Morasso P, Bizzi E, Dichgans J (1973): Adjustment of saccade characteristics during head movements. *Exp Brain Res* 16:492–500

Fly, Visual System

Kuno Kirschfeld

The visual system of the fly comprises the compound eyes with the ocelli and the optic lobes. Interest in this system concerns problems of physiological optics, photoreception, and the structure and function of neurons.

Physiological optics

Each compound eye of the housefly is composed of 3,000 ommatidia (Fig. 1). The facet lens of each ommatidium projects an image onto the plane of the distal endings of the rhabdomeres, i.e., organelles that contain the visual pigment. Light travels down these structures, which act as wave guides: a geometric optical description is not sufficient to describe their properties. Wave theory analysis has shown that the wave properties of light pose the lower limit to the diameter of the rhabdomeres—if they were any thinner they would become inefficient light absorbers. The distance between rhabdomeres in each ommatidium can not be further reduced because of optical crosstalk.

Because the seven rhabdomeres in every ommatidium of the fly eye are not fused, each looks in a different direction (ommatidium I, Fig. 1). The optical axes of rhabdomeres in different ommatidia are aligned so that seven rhabdomeres from seven ommatidia are parallel to each other, looking toward the same point in the environment (Fig. 1, ommatidia C, D, E, in the section plane). The axons of six of them converge in the first optic ganglion (lamina) and superimpose their signals onto the second-order neurons. This neural superposition eye is a subtle construction to improve the absolute sensitivity of this eye without any loss in angular resolution.

Visual and accessory pigments

In contrast to vertebrate visual pigments, the visual pigment of many invertebrates, including the fly, does not decompose into opsin and the chromophore after the absorption of a light quantum; instead it remains stable in the (alltrans =) metastate, and reisomerization is due to absorption of a second light quantum by the metapigment. In contrast, vertebrates need metabolic energy for reisomerization. Unexpectedly, the chromophore of the fly visual pigment is not retinal but 3-hydroxy-retinal. Hence, the visual pigment is not a rhodopsin but a xanthopsin. Also, in most photoreceptor types of the fly eye the interaction between light and visual pigment does not necessarily occur at the normal (Schiffbase-linked) chromophore, but there is a second chromophore (3-hydroxyretinol) that is capable of absorbing ultraviolet light quanta and transferring energy onto the normal chromophore (sensitization). The consequence is that these receptor cells have, in addition to the sensitivity maximum due to the normal chromophore, a pronounced, usually higher, second maximum in the ultraviolet.

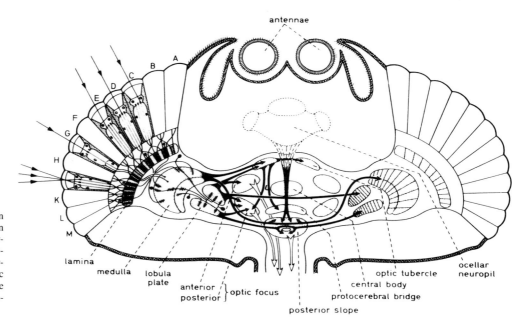

Figure 1. Schematic representation of the visual system of the fly. In several ommatidia (C-E, G, I), cornea lens, crystalline cone, and receptor cells have been drawn. Black arrows indicate projections from optic ganglia to higher order centers of the midbrain; open arrows output projections to the thoracic ganglia.

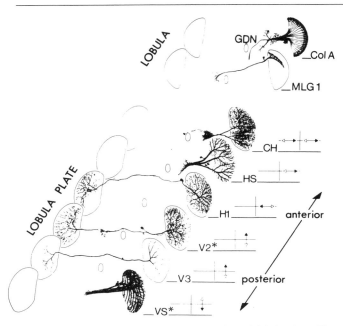

Figure 2. Some giant neurons from the lobula and lobula plate. The margins of both neuropils in the left and right optic lobe are indicated by thin lines. Arrows on the right side indicate the preferred and null directions (filled and open arrowheads, respectively) of the motion-sensitive cells in the lobula plate. Courtesy of K. Hausen.

An advantage of sensitizing pigments in photoreceptors is that the range of spectral sensitivity can be extended over the wavelength scale and the absolute sensitivity increased. In addition to the visual and sensitizing pigments, the rhabdomeres of one class of cells have a third pigment: a C_{40}-carotenoid that has been identified as xanthophyll (zeaxanthin and lutein). This pigment acts as a light filter and modifies the spectral and polarization sensitivity of the photoreceptors. It also helps to solve one problem photoreceptors are confronted with: the deleterious effects of photooxidation. The protective mechanism involves absorption of the most dangerous short wavelength quanta of light and inactivation of activated states of pigments and oxygen (singlet oxygen) by "quenching." This function of C_{40}-carotenoids is equivalent to their function in green plant cells. The pigments in the macula lutea of the human eye are also xanthophylls, and their function most likely is also protective.

Optic lobes

Each optic lobe is composed of three optic ganglia: the lamina, the medulla, and the lobula complex, or lobula and lobula plate (Fig. 1). The interest in a detailed structural study of these ganglia is stimulated primarily by the fact that many of the neurons in these ganglia are large enough to be accessible to a functional analysis by direct electrophysiological techniques.

The basic organization of all three ganglia is retinotopic, i.e., they are composed of the same number of repetitive subunits as are ommatidia in the compound eyes, and also relative

spatial relationships are maintained. The subunits in the lamina are called cartridges; those in the medulla and the lobula complex, columns. Initially there is considerable divergence, each point in the eye is represented by at least six neurons in the lamina and 40 in the medulla. From the medulla to the lobula complex output there is considerable convergence and the retinotopy eventually is lost in higher order centers of the brain.

Within the lamina 12 different neuron types have been described along with their synaptic interconnections. However, it is only possible to record routinely from the two largest ones which both respond with graded potentials. According to these results the main function of the lamina is a kind of gain control: Over the day the receptors have to deal with changes of light intensities that cover a range of many decades, whereas the intensity ratio between bright and dark objects that have to be analyzed simultaneously is usually below 1:10. The lamina, together with the receptors, adjust the working point of the system in such a way that the simultaneously analyzed intensity levels are matched to the dynamic range of some 70 mV of the second-order neurons, irrespective of the mean intensity level.

The function of the lamina *is* hence not to abstract relevant features from the incoming signals. Abstraction processes of this kind seem to be the main function of the medulla. One kind of information extracted by medullar neurons is that of motion of objects in small parts of the visual field. This can be concluded from intracellular recordings of individual neurons, and also from experiments with deoxyglucose, which selectively marks active neurons. Such neurons can be selective or nonselective for the direction of movements. In one type, the change of direction of movement is the significant parameter.

Considerable functional and anatomical details are known from giant neurons of the lobula complex, mainly those of the lobula plate. Anatomy shows that these neurons are uniquely identifiable, usually one type of giant neuron is present once only in each half of the brain, and they are easy to recognize (Fig. 2). Electrophysiology has shown that they are specialized for the detection of relative movement between animal and optical surround (large field movement detectors), and evidence is accumulating that they mediate different kinds of optically induced motor activity. For instance, specific groups of these giant fibers are activated by lift, others by thrust or sideslip, and still others by yaw, roll, or pitch. This information is used to compensate for passive drifts during flight and also probably for object fixation, tracking, and figure-ground discrimination. Such uniquely identifiable giant neurons, only rarely found in vertebrates, are represented not only in the visual system of flies but are common in invertebrate central nervous systems in general.

Further reading

Ali MA, ed. (1984): *Photoreception and Vision in Invertebrates.* New York: Plenum Press

Kirschfeld K (1979): The visual system of the fly: Physiological optics and functional anatomy as related to behavior. In: *The Neurosciences: Fourth Study Program*, Schmitt FO, Worden FG, eds. Cambridge: MIT Press

Fly, Visually Induced Behavior

Werner Reichardt

Complex systems, like the visual system, have many components. A determination of detailed functions is unnecessary for an analysis on a macroscopic scale, such as the behavior of an organism in its environment.

There are three levels of analyzing and understanding complex systems. At the strictly phenomenological level, the overall function, the input-output behavior of the system, and its logical organization are investigated. At the second level the functional principles of the subsystems are the object of the analysis. At the third level, the individual neuronal components and the detailed circuitry are studied.

A phenomenological theory of the fly's visual orientation behavior is sketched here. The theory describes and predicts, at the first level, a rather complex behavior in terms of some simple computations performed by neuronal interactions on V the visual input. At the second level the functional properties of interactions underlying the computations are derived. These two levels of analysis comprise more than just single-cell recordings or histology. A brief outline at the cellular level, from recent investigations of figure-ground and pattern discrimination by the visual system of the fly follows.

Fixation and tracking control system

Male and female flies fixate, that is fly toward small, contrasted patterns, and they track moving objects. The analysis of this visual control system relied almost completely on experiments performed with the flight simulator device shown in Figure 1, which simulates visual input under free-flight conditions in one degree of freedom, rotation around the vertical axis. Results obtained with the device can and have been extended to free-flight conditions.

The flight dynamics of the fly is approximated by the following equation:

$$\theta\ddot{\alpha}_f(t) + k\dot{\alpha}_f(t) = F(t) \qquad (1)$$

where α_f designates the instantaneous direction of flight with respect to an arbitrary zero direction. θ and k are the moment of inertia and an aerodynamic friction constant of the fly, respectively. If α_p designates the instantaneous angular position of an object in the fly's environment, then $\psi = \alpha_p - \alpha_f$ represents the error angle of location of the image of the object on the fly's retina at instant t. Equation (1) can then be rewritten as

$$\theta\ddot{\psi}(t) + k\dot{\psi}(t) = -F(t) + S(t),$$
$$\text{with } S(t) = \theta\ddot{\alpha}_p(t) + k\,\dot{\alpha}_p(t) \qquad (2)$$

where $S(t)$ reflects the trajectory of a moving object relative to the fly. Thus, the fly controls its angular velocity through its own torque F. The basic problem was to determine how F depends on the visual input. A large series of experiments has led to the following conclusions: (1) The observed torque

process is stationary. (2) The term $F(t)$ can be approximated as the sum of two terms: a visually evoked response $R_t\{\psi(s)\}$, representing a functional of the error angle history, and a component that can be characterized stochastically as a Gaussian process $N(t)$, consequently $F(t) = R_t + N(t)$. (3) It has been shown that R_t may be approximated by a function of $\psi(t)$ and its first derivative, given by

$$R_t = D(\psi) + r(\psi) \cdot \dot{\psi}(t) \qquad (3)$$

The terms $D(\psi)$ and $r(\psi)\cdot\dot{\psi}$ have been experimentally determined. $D(\psi)$ carries the position information, whereas $r(\psi)\cdot\dot{\psi}$ is the contribution of a velocity computation. Through Equations (2) and (3) the theory can predict nontrivial behavior in quantitative detail. In a stochastic sense Equations (2) and (3) predict the angular trajectory of a fly's fixating or tracking patterns.

Although connections with physiological and anatomical data are established, the theory is entirely based on behavioral data. Equations (2) and (3) imply that the control system, used by the fly, relies on computations performed on the visual input (extracting movement information and position information), and it states how this information is used to control the flight trajectory.

The phenomenological theory outlined here is restricted to one degree of dynamic freedom, the rotation around the vertical axis of the fly. The vertical degree of freedom, involving the

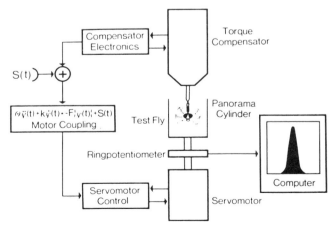

Figure 1. Simplified scheme of the basic closed-loop flight simulator. A fly, fixed to the torque compensator, controls the velocity of a surrounding panorama by its own torque signal through an analog simulation of the flight dynamic. Some of the experiments, for instance, on figure-ground discrimination, have been carried out under open-loop conditions; that is, the movement of the panorama cylinder(s) are controlled by the experimenter, and the torque of a test fly is recorded.

fly's lift, can be described by an equation similar to Equations (2) and (3). It has also been shown that the two degrees of freedom are, with respect to the position response, essentially independent. The results allow a quantitative description of fixation and tracking behavior in two degrees of freedom. Indeed, one would like to extend this analysis to all six degrees of freedom. For instance, the description of translations involves nonlinear terms, arising from the geometry of the situation. This can lead, in their interplay with the control system of the fly, to a complex series of fixation and tracking behaviors.

This analysis of visually guided movements in insects offers a good example of the understanding one can achieve at the highest level of behavioral organization. The analysis considers the logical organization of a specific control system; it neglects explicit computational analysis since the goal of the system is clearly tracking and fixation, provided by modules for movement and position extraction.

Algorithmic specification of neuronal interactions

The phenomenological theory characterizes the basic logical organization of flight behavior controlled by the optical environment. The theory, however, does not specify the interaction, because the variables ψ and $\dot{\psi}$ are only indirectly related to the organization of the receptor inputs and to the interaction processes in the visual nervous system. The theory requires the processing of optical information in the neural network between the receptors and the flight muscles to perform two main computations on the visual input. One computation extracts movement information—the term $r(\psi) \cdot \dot{\psi}$—from the phenomenological Equations (2) and (3); the other provides position information—the term $D(\psi)$.

Algorithm for directionally selective movement computation. If a system or an interaction is movement selective, it must show an average, direction-selective response. The computation of movement requires that the system has at least two light receptor inputs for representing the vector of movement. The property of direction selectivity forces us to assume that the interaction between signals taken up by the receptors is

antisymmetric. Many experiments imply that the algorithm for directional movement detection can be characterized in terms of two input systems with multiplication-like interactions. A graph of the interaction is represented in Figure 2a.

Algorithm for position computation. A system can be said to detect a small contrasted object moving against a white background if its time-averaged output depends on the position of the object in front of the system's photoreceptors. Experiments have shown that the position-dependent part of the time-averaged yaw-torque of the fly does not depend on the light phase, indicating that one-receptor flicker detectors distributed homogeneously in the eye play a fundamental role in this computation. A graph for the most probable interaction responsible for position computation is shown in Figure 2b.

Algorithm for relative-movement computation. Relative movement computation has not been explicitly treated in connection with the phenomenological description, expressed by Equation (2), but should briefly be described here at the algorithmic level. A system can be said to detect relative movement if its average output depends on the position of a visual object moving relative to a larger background, irrespective of its texture. A paradigmatic experiment consists of oscillating an object in front of a textured background that is moving with respect to the fly's array of photoreceptors. In the absence of relative movement, the object disappears in the texture. Relative movement allows a determination of the object's location and, in the fly's case, induces an attempt to fixate it. In a paradigmatic experiment figure (object) and ground are oscillated with the same frequency. The outcome of the experiment depends on the relative phase ϕ between the oscillations. The fly, of course, does not see the object when $\phi = 0°$. However, it reacts strongly when $\phi = 90°$ or $270°$. Interestingly, it does not react to the object when $\psi = 180°$. The phase portrait is well approximated at this oscillation frequency by the time averaged response

$$\bar{R} = k_0(\omega) - k_4(\omega) \cos(2 \cdot \phi) \qquad (4)$$

which speaks in favor of an algorithm whose graphic representation is pictured in Figure 2c.

Cellular basis of figure-ground discrimination and pattern discrimination

A model of the neuronal circuitry for figure-ground discrimination via relative movement by the visual system of the fly has been proposed. Two results have been obtained: (1) The characteristic properties of figure-ground discrimination are observed not only under binocular but also under monocular stimulation by the ground. (2) The torque response of the fly follows the oscillation of a given pattern. Experiments have shown that the amplitude of the response increases with increasing movement amplitude (pattern speed), whereas it is almost independent of the dimensions of the pattern, suggesting a specific gain control mechanism. These and other findings have led to a proposal for a neuronal circuit obeying the following constraints: The circuit should contain a gain control mechanism for the overall optomotor reaction. The interaction between movement detectors is not realized through a lateral inhibitory network but through large-field movement-selective neurons inhibiting elementary movement detectors.

A model for the neuronal circuitry satisfying these constraints is shown in Figure 3. The model has two properties required by experimental evidence: (1) The gain control property of the optomotor response makes the response to a moving

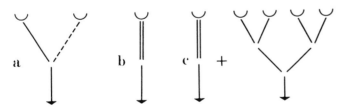

Figure 2. Graphic representations of algorithms for movement, position, and relative movement computations.
a. Movement computation. The graphic representation of the algorithm pictures a system (module) with two receptor inputs and an antisymmetric, multiplication-like interaction (expressed by a dotted line). b. Position computation. The graph of the algorithm represents a system (module) with one receptor input and a multiplication-like interaction that ensures a time-averaged response when an object is moved across the receptor input. The system is parametrized in the sense that its response is dependent on the location of the position-detector in the compound eye. c. Relative movement computation. The graphic representation of the system consists of two modules. The one on the left represents a position-detector, the other a combination of three movement detectors with multiplication-like interactions, measuring the cross-coherency of the directionally independent movement signals. The graph on the right has four receptor inputs and is therefore double orientation specific.

Figure 3. Outline of the model circuitry for figure-ground and pattern discrimination for the right and left compound eye. If the right eye is used as an example, two retinotopic arrays of elementary movement detectors, responding selectively to progressive (—▶) and regressive (◀—) motion serve as input channels to the neural circuitry. The two arrays share the same field of view. They are drawn apart from each other. A pool neuron (S_R) summates the movement detector outputs (—◀ indicates excitatory synapses) as well as the input from its contralateral homolog (S_L). Its output is assumed to undergo a saturation effect (modeled by taking the square root of its overall excitation; $q = 0.5$) and to shunt inhibit each movement detector channel via presynaptic inhibition. The synapses involved (—△) should therefore inhibit (opening ionic channels with an equilibrium battery close to the resting potential) the output of each elementary detector channel. The cell X_R summates the progressive (excitatory—●◀) and regressive (inhibitory—◯◁) detectors. Progressive channels have a higher amplification than regressive ones. The synapses on the X-cell are assumed to operate with a nonlinear input-output characteristic, leading to postsynaptic signals that are approximately the square ($n = 2$) of the inputs. The motor output is controlled by the X-cells via a direct channel and a channel T computing the running average of X-cell output. According to the circuitry, the behavioral response is given by the relation, $R = Nx^n/[\beta + (Nx)^q]^n$, except for the running average at the output and provided that all channels N are equally excited by a moving pattern. x designates the output of each of the N movement detectors and β the shunting inhibition coefficient.

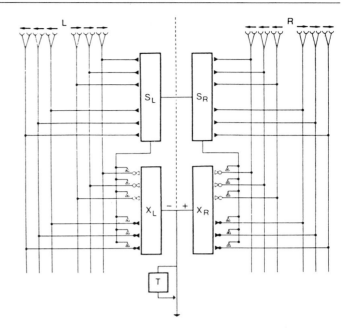

object or figure independent of its angular size. (2) Object or figure and ground are independently detected when they move in statistical independence.

More recent experimental and theoretical investigations have shown that pattern discrimination by the fly is a special (degenerate) case of the figure-ground discrimination system described in Figure 3. The output of movement detectors depends not only on pattern velocity, but also on contrast, average brightness, and other pattern parameters. These properties determine the pattern discrimination properties of the fly, as well as other insects.

These experiments attempted to design a cellular topology, derived from quantitative, behavioral experiments. Cellular components must, of course be determined directly by histology and electrophysiology in order to associate real nerve cells to the topological structure outlined in Figure 3. Extensive investigations have been carried out at the level of the third optical ganglion (*lobula plate*) where large neurons integrate

the output signals of large arrays of movement detectors. Specifically it has been shown that neuronal correlates of the output cells of the model circuitry, shown in Figure 3, are located in the lobula plate. These output cells can be subdivided into two classes with different spatial integration properties. One of them is more sensitive to large field pattern stimulation; the other responds best to the motion of small patterns (objects).

Further reading

Reichardt W (1979): Functional characterization of neural interactions through an analysis of behaviour. In: *The Neurosciences: Fourth Study Program*, Schmitt FO, Worden FG eds. Cambridge: MIT Press

Reichardt W, Poggio T (1976): Visual control of orientation behaviour in the fly. *Q Rev Biophys* 9:311–375

Reichardt W, Poggio T, Hausen K (1983): Figure-ground discrimination by relative movement. *Biol Cybernet* 46(Suppl):1–30

Gaze, Control of

Reuben S. Gellman and Frederick A. Miles

For optimal visual acuity, images on the retina should be reasonably stable and those of particular interest should be located centrally where receptors are most densely distributed. These needs are met by the oculomotor system, which prevents excessive disturbances of the image and can rapidly reposition the eyes to bring new images into the central retina. Many frontal-eyed animals possess stereovision for which the oculomotor system must be able to direct both eyes at the same object.

The major potential threat to the stability of the retinal image of the world is head movement, and both visual and nonvisual mechanisms are employed to minimize this problem. Nonvisual stabilization uses information from end organs that sense accelerations of the head. Rotational accelerations are sensed, in vertebrates, by the semicircular canals whose signals are used to generate compensatory eye movements that offset the rotation of the head and thereby stabilize gaze in space (the dynamic vestibulo-ocular reflex). Linear accelerations are sensed by the otolith organs that signal orientation of the head with respect to gravity. These signals are used to counterroll the eyes during static head tilt (the static vestibulo-ocular reflex). In many animals, including humans and monkeys, the static reflex is not very effective.

Visual stabilization mechanisms, often referred to as the optokinetic response, are brought into operation when short-comings in the nonvisual mechanisms result in retinal image slip. In the laboratory these mechanisms are studied by moving the visual scene. If prolonged, this leads to nystagmus, a pattern of alternating slow and quick movements, the former tracking the scene and the latter, known as quick phases, resetting the eyes when they become excessively deviated. Similarly rapid eye movements, known as saccadic eye movements, are used to transfer fixation between objects of interest, their high speed minimizing the duration of the attendant visual disturbance. If the object of fixation should move, even against a stationary featured background, some animals can use the smooth pursuit tracking system to keep the retinal image centered.

For stereovision, the two lines of sight must converge on the same object, which can vary in its distance from the observer, necessitating vergence eye movements. These disjunctive movements are very slow, and are driven mainly by retinal disparity with some contribution from other depth cues such as blur.

Further reading

Carpenter RHS (1977): *Movements of the Eyes*. London: Pion

Leigh JL, Zee DS (1983): *The Neurology of Eye Movements*. Philadelphia: Davis

Gaze, Plasticity in the Control of

Frederick A. Miles and Reuben S. Gellman

In order for visual exploration of the environment to proceed efficiently, gaze must be controlled with precision. In vertebrates, the different movements of the eyes are the result of processing in several relatively independent subsystems within the brain, each of which relies on visually mediated learning mechanisms to achieve an appropriate input-output relationship, or gain. In order to ascertain whether a particular parameter of oculomotor behavior is plastic, i.e., subject to adaptive gain control, a disturbance must be introduced into the control loop to render the current value of the parameter in question inappropriate. This has commonly been done with a reversible, noninvasive optical challenge, tailor-made to stress only the parameter of interest; the system's adaptive capability is then assessed from its ability to compensate. Most of this work has been carried out on primates—both human and nonhuman—but there have also been important studies on cats, rabbits, and fish. Additional evidence has come from studying the human patient's ability to compensate for various oculomotor disorders. Many of the adaptive mechanisms in the oculomotor system are known to be compromised by damage to the cerebellum, but the exact nature of its role in these processes is at present unclear.

Saccadic eye movements

The saccadic system rapidly redirects the eyes toward eccentric targets of interest. Contact lenses magnify (or reduce) the visual images and so alter their eccentricity on the retina, thereby altering the input error seen by the saccadic system. In the laboratory, this effect has been simulated by consistently shifting the target while the subject is in the act of trying to acquire it with a saccade. Provided that the shift is not too large the subject does not even perceive it. Depending on the nature of the shift, subjects at first consistently under- or overshoot the target with their primary saccades and must follow up with unusually large secondary correctives. However, subjects soon begin to compensate and in minutes are acquiring the displaced targets with their primary saccades with customary accuracy. The saccadic system can also compensate for more profound dysmetrias, such as those that result from weakness of the extraocular muscles, but here the adaptive processes require days for completion.

The vestibulo-ocular reflex

Ordinarily, the retinal image of the surrounding world is kept reasonably stable during head turns by counter rotations of the eyes that are produced primarily by the vestibulo-ocular reflex (VOR). Magnifying (or reducing) telescopic spectacles selectively increase (or decrease) the magnitude of the eye movements required to compensate for any given head rotation and have been shown to induce appropriate increases (or de-

creases) in the gain of the VOR. (Note that these spectacles move with the head and—unlike contact lenses—not with the eyes, so that they do not interfere with the operation of the saccadic system.) While the system may take several days to compensate for the extreme challenge of these telescopic spectacles, the more modest stress of spectacles such as those ordinarily used for reading can be fully compensated in less than an hour.

Left-right reversing prisms present a much more complex challenge to the adaptive mechanisms protecting this reflex: in addition to reversing the visual input associated with horizontal (yaw) rotations of the head (stressing the horizontal VOR), they also reverse the visual input associated with rolling the head from side to side (stressing the torsional VOR), but do not alter the visual input associated with pitch rotations of the head (which stimulate the vertical VOR). The nervous system is able to respond appropriately to this asymmetrical optical challenge, selectively attenuating the compensatory eye movements associated with rotations about the yaw and roll axes while leaving those concerned with rotations about the pitch axis unaffected. Such specificity is one of the hallmarks of the adaptive mechanisms in the oculomotor system.

Visual tracking

One major function of visual tracking is to help stabilize the eyes with respect to the stationary surroundings. The need for such tracking occurs most commonly during head turns when the VOR fails to provide compensatory eye movements that are of exactly the right magnitude. Primates, if they so choose, can also track small targets that move across the stationary background. If the gain of such tracking systems is too low, their responses are sluggish and the eyes tend to lag far behind the target of interest. On the other hand, if the gain is too high, responses are much more brisk but the eyes tend to overshoot the target and may even oscillate around it. Normally, these systems have a gain that represents a compromise between these two extremes, so that responses are reasonably brisk yet free of any tendency to oscillate, and this is the result of visually mediated adaptive mechanisms. This has been demonstrated experimentally using a visual display moved under computer control: When retinal events similar to those that might be expected to prevail when the gain is clearly too low (undershoot) or too high (overshoot) are induced artificially, the system is able to compensate appropriately. In the cases examined, compensation required several days for completion.

Vergence and accommodation

The transfer of fixation between targets that are at different distances from the observer raises two additional problems:

to maintain correct focus—and hence clear vision—the focal power of the eye lens must be adjusted (accommodation), and to maintain binocular alignment—and hence single vision—appropriate vergence eye movements must be executed. Accommodation and vergence are each subject to independent, negative feedback control. However, there are cross-links between these two systems, mediating the so-called accommodative vergence and vergence accommodation responses. In normal binocular viewing conditions, accommodation and vergence operate in concert, and the parameter that determines the strength of the desired link between them is a geometric factor, the separation of the two eyes: the greater the separation, the greater the required change in vergence per unit change in accommodation. Increasing the effective separation of the two lines of sight by means of laterally displacing periscopic spectacles has been shown to cause appropriate adaptive changes in both the accommodative vergence and vergence accommodation responses—increases and decreases, respectively. Thirty minutes were sufficient to elicit 50% changes.

Contact lenses alter the amount of accommodation required to produce sharp retinal images of the object of regard without affecting the vergence angle required for its binocular alignment. Positive lenses, for example, reduce the amount of accommodation required to focus the eyes for any given viewing distance; this immediately leads to an increase in the amount of convergence associated with any given level of accommodation. If such lenses are left in place for a few minutes, this extra convergence persists (as an esophoria) even in the monocular viewing situation. Medially or laterally displacing wedge prisms have the converse effect insofar as they affect the vergence angle required for binocular alignment on any given object but do not affect the amount of accommodation required to produce focused retinal images of it. Base-out prisms, for example, increase the required vergence angle associated with fixation targets at any given distance. Like positive lenses, base-out prisms lead to an increase in the amount of convergence associated with any given level of accommodation and again this extra convergence persists as an esophoria during monocular testing. It is important to realize that the effect of lenses and wedge prisms is independent of viewing distance, while the effect of periscopic spectacles is in inverse relation to the viewing distance. Thus, studies on the cross coupling between the vergence and accommodation control systems have successfully used lenses and wedge prisms to reveal adaptive mechanisms regulating the offset in the linkage between the two, and laterally displacing periscopes to reveal that the gain of the linkage is also subject to adaptive regulation.

Further reading

Leigh JL, Zee DS (1983): *The Neurology of Eye Movements*. Philadelphia: Davis

Miles FA (1983): Plasticity in the transfer of gaze. *Trends Neurosci* 6:57–60

Miles FA, Lisberger SG (1981): Plasticity in the vestibulo-ocular reflex: A new hypothesis. *Annu Rev Neurosci* 4:273–299

Geniculate Body, Lateral

Pedro Pasik and Tauba Pasik

The geniculate bodies are nuclear masses belonging to the dorsal thalamus that have detached from it during ontogeny and are therefore designated as the metathalamus. They comprise two major structures: the lateral geniculate nucleus (LGN) related to the visual system, and the medial geniculate nucleus, a part of the auditory system. The lateral geniculate nucleus has two components: the pars dorsalis (LGNd) and the pars ventralis (LGNv).

LGNd

The LGNd is usually a layered structure. In the primate, the laminae are numbered 1–6 from ventral to dorsal (Fig. 1). Laminae 1 and 2 are magnocellular, i.e., large-celled, and 3–6 are parvocellular, i.e., small-celled. The LGNd is the site of termination of most, if not all, optic tract fibers. These axons originate in the temporal half of the ipsilateral retina and in the nasal half of the contralateral retina, except that a narrow strip on each side of the vertical meridian supplies both optic tracts. The inputs from the ipsilateral and contralateral eye remain segregated in laminae 2, 3, and 5, and 1, 4, and 6, respectively. An additional pair of layers (S laminae) has also been described in a location ventral to lamina 1. It is possible that laminae 3 and 5, and 4 and 6 represent leaflets of single parvocellular layers receiving ipsilateral and contralateral input, respectively. Besides the fibers of retinal origin, the LGNd receives a large contingent of fibers from the visual cerebral cortex originating in cortical layer VI and other structures such as the thalamic reticular nucleus, and superior colliculus. Finally, serotoninergic innervation is provided by the dorsal raphe nuclei, noradrenergic input by the locus ceruleus.

The LGNd laminae contain two categories of neurons: principal long-axoned cells (P cells), which project mostly to the striate cortex or area 17, and to a minor extent to area 18, and interneurons (I cells) with intrinsic axons. Morphological classifications of neuronal types based on Golgi impregnations have been questioned because neurons driven antidromically from the cortex, thence P cells, and visualized by the histochemical reaction product of intracellularly injected horseradish peroxidase, showed features attributed to I cells in Golgi material. The two types, however, are quite distinct ultrastructurally in the monkey LGNd. The P cells, which show signs of acute retrograde degeneration days after total ablation of visual cortex, and completely disappear after several months, are characterized by a centrally located, smooth nucleus, cytoplasm rich in all organelles including large, medium-dense mitochondria. The I cells, which remain intact after cortical excisions, have eccentric, deeply invaginated nuclei, cytoplasm poor in organelles with small dense mitochondria and clusters of synaptic vesicles. The mitochondrial type and the absence or presence of synaptic vesicles also help in differentiating the dendritic elements of these two cell types within the neuropil. The I

cell population is more numerous in the magnocellular layers (15–16% of the total) than in the parvocellular layers (4–5% of the total).

A characteristic property of the I cell is that the membrane may become presynaptic not only in the axonal terminals, but also in any and all regions of the neuron, i.e., the perikaryon, proximal and distal dendrites, axon hillock, and axon initial segment. The presynaptic character of I cell dendrites, which are also postsynaptic in accordance with their dendritic nature, gives rise to complex synaptic arrangements of the triadic, serial, and reciprocal types. The most common one is the triadic synapse (Fig. 2) where a retinal terminal is presynaptic to both a P cell dendrite and an I cell dendrite, the latter being presynaptic to the same P cell dendrite. Axonal terminals of cortical origin can also serve as input elements to triadic arrangements in lieu of the retinal axons. Finally, ample connectivity between I cells is also present. Little is known of the synaptic connections of other afferents to the LGNd.

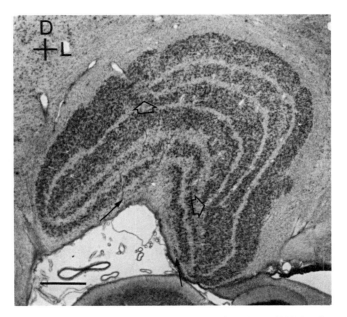

Figure 1. Coronal section through the middle of monkey LGNd showing the organization of cell laminae (dark bands). The two ventral magnocellular laminae (1 and 2) and the four dorsal parvocellular laminae (3–6) are self-evident. Note also the areas of continuity between laminae 3 and 5, and 4 and 6 indicated by open arrows, and the thin laminae S (arrows). D, dorsal; L, lateral. Cresyl violet stain. Scale: 1 mm (corrected for shrinkage).

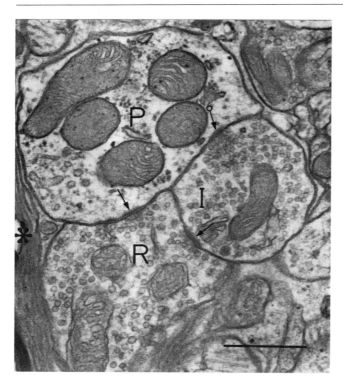

Figure 2. Triadic arrangement characteristic of LGNd synaptic organization. Retinal terminal (R) is presynaptic at arrows to a P cell dendrite (P) and an I cell dendrite (I). The I cell dendrite, in turn, is presynaptic at ringed arrow to the same P cell dendrite. Partial glial wrappings indicated by asterisk. Scale: 0.5 μm.

The neurotransmitters involved in the synaptic transactions at the LGNd have been only partially identified. Gamma-aminobutyric acid (GABA) is a prominent inhibitory substance that is present in I cells and also in axon terminals originating in the thalamic reticular nucleus. Glutamate is apparently the transmitter in cortical terminals. Serotoninergic boutons, forming synapses with both I and P cell dendrites, have also been visualized. The issue of neurotransmitters in retinal terminals is unresolved, but several amino acids and peptides have been considered.

Electrophysiological recordings have defined the receptive field characteristics of geniculate neurons. Many of the features of P cells are shared with retinal ganglion cells. A center-surround antagonistic organization is present, with center on and center off neurons predominating in laminae 5–6 and 3–4, respectively. Parvocellular laminae, which receive the bulk of the input from the central visual fields via axons of X-type retinal ganglion cells, are almost exclusively made of X cells and include color-opponent neurons, i.e., one color excites the center and another inhibits the surround of the receptive field, and vice-versa. Their terminal axonal arborization occurs in layers 4A and 4C beta of the striate cortex. Magnocellular laminae, where most of the peripheral fields project via axons of Y-type retinal ganglion cells, have a mixed population of Y cells and X cells. Y cells respond well to rapid stimulus movement and do not exhibit color opponency. Their axons terminate in layer 4C alpha of the striate cortex. The S laminae apparently receive axons of the W group of retinal ganglion cells. There is some evidence in the cat that triadic synapses made by retinal terminals and interneuron presynaptic dendrites are established more frequently with X cells than with Y cell principal dendrites.

Contrary to retinal ganglion cells, geniculate neurons do not respond at all to diffuse illumination, and the probability of firing increases with decreasing stimulus size. In spite of the segregated inputs from the two eyes, some binocular interaction can be recorded from the geniculate neurons in the form of inhibition on stimulating the retina which does not project to the recorded lamina. This interaction can be accomplished through P cell dendrites extending into an adjacent lamina, as noted in the magnocellular division, or through I cell dendrites crossing laminar borders as seen particularly in the parvocellular segment.

The understanding of information processing at the geniculate level has been aided by the construction of mathematical models. One such model has proposed that the coupling of triadic synapses by means of a common presynaptic dendrite gives rise to different discharge patterns of a given P cell according to the size and velocity of the stimulus. Moreover, the degree of synchrony of various stimuli may be sensed by further coupling of triads through serial synapses between interneurons, which introduces a certain degree of anisotropy in the system.

LGNv. This structure is also called the pregeniculate nucleus in the primate (not to be confused with the cat perigeniculate nucleus). It is a small but rather complex nucleus which includes several subunits. It receives topologically arranged afferents from the retina of both eyes (mostly from W-type ganglion cells), the superior colliculus, the visual cortex, and probably pretectal nuclei and the LGNd as well. The efferents do not project to the cortex but to several subcortical structures that in addition receive retinal afferents, namely, pretectal nuclei, superior colliculus, nucleus of the accessory optic tract, and suprachiasmatic nuclei. A projection to the zona incerta has also been described. Many neurons of the LGNv are GABA-immunoreactive. GABAergic axon terminals are also heavily represented in the neuropil.

The receptive fields of LGNv neurons differ from those of the LGNd in that they are of greater variety and extent and many are binocularly driven. The LGNv has been implicated in the pupillary light reflex, visually guided saccadic eye movements, and a centrifugal system influencing vision at central structures instead of at the retinal level as found in nonmammalian species.

Further reading

Bishop PO (1984): Processing of visual information within the retinostriate system. In: *Handbook of Physiology, the Nervous System, Vol III, Sensory Processes.* Darian-Smith I, ed. Baltimore: Williams and Wilkins

Hámori J, Pasik P, Pasik T (1983): Differential frequency of P-cells and I-cells in magnocellular and parvocellular laminae of monkey lateral geniculate nucleus. An ultrastructural study. *Exp Brain Res* 52:57–66

Lábos E (1977): Theoretical considerations of local neuron circuits and their triadic synaptic arrangements (TSA) in subcortical sensory nuclei. *J Neurosci Res* 3:1–10

Spear PD, Smith DC, Williams LL (1977): Visual receptive field properties of single neurons in cat's ventral lateral geniculate nucleus. *J Neurophysiol* 40:390–409

Stone J, Dreher B, Leventhal A (1979): Hierarchical and parallel mechanisms in the organization of visual cortex. *Brain Res Rev* 1:345–394

Imagery, Mental

Stephen M. Kosslyn

Historically, the term mental image has been used ambiguously, either to refer to the internal representation that gives rise to the experience of perceiving in the absence of the appropriate sensory input, or to the conscious experience of "seeing with the mind's eye" (or "hearing with the mind's ear," and so on). In contemporary scientific psychology, the term is used to refer to the internal representation that gives rise to the percept-like experience, not to the conscious experience itself. This internal representation is taken to correspond to a particular brain state. It is assumed that this brain state gives rise (somehow) to the conscious experience; thus, the experience of "having a mental image" is a hallmark that the underlying imagery brain state is present.

What is imagery for?

As our characterization of imagery implies, there is a close relationship between imagery and perception. This relationship has been explored most deeply for visual imagery and perception, where the uses of imagery to some extent parallel those of perception. That is, we use vision primarily for two different purposes: First, we use it to attempt to recognize objects and their parts. Second, we use vision to navigate as we move through space (and not bump into things or step into pits) and to track moving objects (avoiding or intercepting them, as is appropriate). Similarly, one purpose of imagery is to recognize properties of imaged objects, allowing us to access information stored in memory. For example, consider how you answer the following questions: What shape are a beagle's ears? Which is darker green, a Christmas tree or a frozen pea? Which is bigger, a tennis ball or a 100-watt light bulb? Most people claim that they visualize the objects and "look" at them in order to answer these questions, and the behavioral data support this claim. Imagery is most often used in memory retrieval when the information to be remembered is a subtle visual property that has not been explicitly considered previously and cannot be easily deduced from other facts (e.g., about the object's category in general).

Another function of imagery parallels our perceptual mapping and tracking abilities: Imagery is a way of anticipating what would happen if we moved in a particular way or something else moved relative to us. For example, we might imagine a jar and "see" if there is room for it on the top refrigerator shelf; or we might mentally project an object's trajectory, "seeing" where it will come to rest. Thus, imagery is also used when we reason about visual appearances of objects under transformation, especially when subtle visual relations are involved.

Finally, we are able to use these imagery abilities in the service of more abstract thinking and learning. Shepard and Cooper review cases of scientific problem solving in which "imaged models" were used as aids to reasoning. Einstein, for example, claimed that his first insight into relativity came when he imagined himself chasing a beam of light and "saw" what it looked like when he finally matched its speed. In addition, images of objects or events can themselves be encoded into memory, which improves retention of the material.

The nature of imagery

Most research on imagery has focused on its functional properties. This literature can be organized into several classes.

Shared perceptual mechanisms. Although the uses of imagery to some extent parallel those of like-modality perception, this similarity does not necessarily imply that the same neural mechanisms are used in both cases. However, there is good evidence that imagery does in fact recruit mechanisms specialized for processing in a specific sensory modality. This inference is based in part on findings that imagery selectively interferes with like-modality perception. For example, S.J. Segal and V. Fusella found that maintaining a visual image impairs visual perception more than auditory perception, but maintaining an auditory image has the reverse effects. R.A. Finke reports numerous results that suggest that imagery uses "central" perceptual mechanisms.

Image/percept analogs. In many ways, imaged objects behave like actual objects that are being watched. For example, the time to rotate an object in a mental image increases with the amount the object is rotated, as would happen if an actual object were rotated. This finding is remarkable because images are not actual objects that must obey the laws of physics. Because velocity cannot be instantaneous, real objects must pass through intermediate points along the trajectory as they change orientation; but images are not real objects. Rather, it appears that our imagery mechanisms are built so that imaged events are constrained to mimic actual physical events. Indeed, the process of "looking" at objects in images mirrors actual perception in many ways. For example, the time subjects require to "see" parts of imaged objects increases when objects are imagined at smaller rather than at larger sizes. This result suggests that objects in images are subject to spatial summation, and objects must be imagined at larger sizes if the details are to be apparent (subjects typically claim that they have to "zoom in" to see parts of objects imagined at a small size). Similarly, the time to scan across an imaged object or scene increases linearly with the distance scanned. S. Pinker found that time to scan is determined by the distance in three dimensions, although subjects can be induced to scan across the two-dimensional projection in the picture plane.

Learning and memory. Objects are remembered better than words. Thus, it is not surprising that if we can image the referent of a word, the word will be learned and remembered better than if the referent is an abstract entity (e.g., ''justice''). Indeed, explicitly instructing subjects to use imagery to learn improves memory. However, the kind of image formed is important: For example, G.H. Bower found that pairs of words are recalled better if the named objects are imagined interacting in some way than if they are imaged separated in space. In addition, there is evidence that imagining practicing some activity, such as a gymnastic move or throwing a ball through a hoop, helps one to learn it; however, to be effective such mental practice must be intermixed with actual practice.

Processing system. Another body of work tries to specify the nature of the representations and processes used in imagery; this work tends to be oriented around developments in the field of artificial intelligence and makes use of computer simulation models. Some research of this type has focused on the internal structure of image representations, whereas other research has focused on how images are processed. For example, the way in which images are generated from stored information has been studied in some detail. It has been found that the time to generate a mental image increases linearly with increases in the number of parts making up the imaged object, with ''parts'' being defined both by stimulus properties and by the way a subject tries to organize a pattern. This result suggests that parts are stored individually and activated one at a time when images are formed.

Individual differences. The earliest scientific research on imagery focused on the nature of individual differences. It has been well established that people report differences in the qualities of their imagery. Some researchers find that such reports predict performance in a variety of tasks; for example, D.F. Marks found that people who claimed to have vivid imagery remembered pictures better than those who claimed to have dim imagery. Other researchers have not been successful in using such reports to predict performance. An alternative approach examines individual differences in the performance of objective tasks that require imagery. This approach has revealed that imagery is a collection of subabilities, and skill on each one is only weakly, if at all, correlated with skill on the others.

Imagery and cerebral localization

Imagery is not a unitary, undifferentiated phenomenon. Rather, imagery can be broken down into a number of subabilities, such as the ability to generate images, to inspect them, to transform them, and to maintain them over time. Not all these abilities must be exercised to perform any given task; for example, image transformation abilities need not be used in many memory retrieval tasks (e.g., remembering the way to get to the train station). This observation is important if we are to consider how imagery is carried out in the brain. Imagery is not an exclusively left or right hemisphere phenomenon. Rather, there is evidence from a variety of sources that imagery depends on mechanisms located in various parts of the brain.

Image generation. Brain damage can selectively affect the ability to evoke images of objects from memory. In addition, Farah found that virtually all of the patients who could not generate images had a posterior lesion in the left cerebral hemisphere. This observation is consistent with results from studies of image generation in patients who, for medical reasons, have had corpus callosum transections. In these studies, the left hemisphere was far superior when images had to be composed from separate parts; when images of single forms were all that was necessary to perform the task, both hemispheres performed comparably. This finding supports the idea that image generation itself is not a unitary ability, but rather is carried out by a number of distinct ''processing modules.'' One of these processing modules, it is hypothesized, uses stored descriptions of spatial relationships among parts to arrange them correctly, and this module is typically better developed in the left hemisphere.

Image transformation. There is evidence that at least one component of our image transformation abilities is typically more effective in the right cerebral hemisphere. For example, it has been found that subjects with right parietal lobe damage have difficulty mentally rotating objects or ''mentally folding'' cubes. In addition, it has been found that the isolated right hemisphere of a split brain patient was better than the isolated left hemisphere at performing spatial manipulation tasks. However, other studies have presented a mixed picture, suggesting that at least some image transformation processing is bilateral.

Image inspection. Patients with right parietal lobe damage sometimes show ''unilateral visual neglect''; they ignore objects to their left side. E. Bisiach and C. Luzzatti found that patients who showed such neglect in perception also showed it in imagery, even when they tried to imagine a scene that was very familiar prior to the injury. This result provides additional evidence that the mechanisms responsible for attending to parts of real space are also involved in attending to parts of imagined space, and suggests that the right hemisphere processes a topographic representation of locations in space.

In short, there is evidence that both hemispheres are involved in imagery, with the right parietal lobe having a prominent role in both image transformation and image inspection and the left hemisphere having a prominent role in image generation. The scientific study of the neural substrate of imagery is in its infancy, but we have good reason to suspect that important discoveries will emerge in the near future: Mental imagery has emerged from its status as an inaccessible, private event and is now the subject of intense scientific study.

Further reading

Erlichman H, Barrett J (1983): Right hemisphere specialization for mental imagery: A review of the evidence. *Brain and Cognition* 2:55–76

Farah MJ (1984): The neurological basis of mental imagery: A componential analysis. *Cognition* 18:245–272

Kosslyn SM (1983): *Ghosts in the Mind's Machine.* New York: Norton

Shepard RN, Cooper LA (1982): *Mental Images and Their Transformations.* Cambridge: MIT Press

Nystagmus

Volker Henn

Nystagmus is an involuntary reflex eye movement with a characteristic alternation of slow and rapid movements (Fig. 1). Its function is to stabilize vision. During a head movement, for the eyes to remain fixed on a stationary target, they have to move in the opposite direction. Or if a large visual stimulus moves, to see it unblurred, the eyes move with it. The vestibular (head movement) or visual stimulus moves the eyes and determines their velocity and direction. In the horizontal, vertical, or oblique directions slow phase eye velocity can reach stimulus velocity. Nystagmus is then said to have a gain of unity. For rotatory nystagmus (movement of the stimulus and of the eyes around the line of sight like looking at the center of a rotating wheel), the induced eye movement is much slower than stimulus movement, i.e., the response has a low gain. The stimulus-dependent phase of the nystagmus is called slow phase. As the eyes can move only over a limited angle, there is a quick resetting of the eyes in the opposite direction. Like saccades, this fast phase belongs to the class of rapid eye movements and shares the same neuronal generator.

Vestibular nystagmus is induced by labyrinthine stimulation and is called the vestibulo-ocular reflex (VOR). Optokinetic nystagmus (OKN) is induced by a moving visual stimulus. Optokinetic afternystagmus (OKAN) is the nystagmus outlasting OKN after lights are turned off. A cervico-ocular reflex (COR), in which the trunk moves relative to the body, can also induce nystagmus, although it is frequently absent or very limited in primates. To measure nystagmus quantitatively one determines the velocity of the slow phase and its direction. As the quick phases of nystagmus are so striking, nystagmus direction has traditionally been defined as the direction of its fast phase.

As nystagmus can be induced by different sensory systems, and as it is a reflex response, its observation and measurement in patients is an important part of every clinical examination. Nystagmus is pathological if it does not match stimulus velocity over a certain range. In most instances, it is too slow. Patients might then experience dizziness and blurred vision because of incorrect motion information and because their eyes move too slowly to stabilize vision. Nystagmus can also be too fast. An example is spontaneous nystagmus in the absence of any stimulus. This usually occurs when there is a mismatch of vestibular inputs from the two sides and can reach extreme values in the case of sudden loss of function of one labyrinth. Patients then experience an acute attack of vertigo with spontaneous nystagmus directed away from the affected labyrinth.

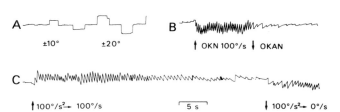

Figure 1. Normal human horizontal nystagmus. A. Calibration of eye position; upward deflection rightward eye movement. B. Optokinetic nystagmus and afternystagmus to the left. The subject sits inside a drum that rotates at 100·/sec to the right; arrows indicate light on and off. C. Vestibular nystagmus to the right in response to a rightward angular acceleration of 100·/sec² to a constant velocity of 100·/sec in total darkness. Upward arrow marks time of acceleration; downward arrow, time of deceleration (rest of recording cut off). From Henn et al (1982): *Human Neurobiol* 1:87–95.

Further reading

Henn V, Cohen B, Young LR (1980): Visual-vestibular interaction in motion perception and the generation of nystagmus. *Neurosci Res Prog Bull* 18:457–651

Henn V, Hepp K, Büttner-Ennever JA (1982): The primate oculomotor system. II Premotor System—a synthesis of anatomical, physiological, and clinical data. *Human Neurobiol* 1:87–95

Robinson DA (1977): Vestibular and optokinetic symbiosis: an example of explaining by modeling. In: *Control of Gaze by Brain Stem Neurons*, Baker R, Berthoz A, eds. Amsterdam: Elsevier-North Holland

Oculomotor System, Mechanisms

Masao Ito

The oculomotor system consists of extraocular muscles attached to the eye ball, motoneurons in the IIIrd (oculomotor), IVth (trochlear), and VIth (abducens) cranial nerve nuclei, and premotor systems. Three pairs of extraocular muscles (medial and lateral rectus, superior and inferior rectus, superior and inferior oblique), each subserving horizontal, vertical, or rotatory eye movement, respectively, conjointly produce an eye movement. Various types of oculomotor activities are distinguished, e.g., fixation, saccade, and slow movement. The same motoneurons participate in all these activities, none of which is the exclusive product of one type of motoneuron. Impulse discharge rates in each motoneuron are represented by the sum of two terms, one proportional to eye position and the other to eye velocity. However, values of the proportion coefficients vary widely among motoneurons, yielding five major types of responses (tonic, predominantly tonic, tonic-phasic, predominantly phasic, and phasic). Since direct application of currents to the motoneuronal membrane elicits tonic discharge with a frequency linearly related to injected currents, the varied responses of motoneurons related to eye movements should reflect mainly the properties of their input signals from premotor systems. Premotor systems provide command signals for execution of varied reflexive and voluntary eye movements.

Ocular reflexes

One of the major inputs to motoneurons for extraocular muscles arises from the vestibular nuclei and mediates the vestibulo-ocular reflex (VOR). The VOR produces eye movements compensatory for head movements so as to secure visual stability during head movements. In this reflex, signals generated from the vestibular labyrinths are forwarded to the vestibular nuclei through the VIIIth nerve, activating VOR relay neurons that in turn either excite or inhibit motoneurons for extraocular muscles. The vestibular labyrinth contains two otolith organs (macula and saccule) and three semicircular canals (lateral, anterior, and posterior), each of which senses gravitational or acceleratory forces in different directions. Accordingly, the VOR is performed by parallel pathways arising from different end organs and terminating at different extraocular muscles. Figure 1 illustrates the component pathway arising from a lateral semicircular canal and ending at the ipsilateral lateral and medial rectus muscles, which subserve horizontal eye movements.

Another representative ocular reflex is the optokinetic response (OKR), which produces eye movement following a slow movement of the visual surroundings. Under stationary visual surroundings, the OKR also acts to stabilize eye position; otherwise, there will be continuous drifting and rapid resetting of eye movements. The OKR is initiated by visual signals mediated by the nucleus reticularis tegmenti pontis, which projects to vestibular nuclei, directly in rabbits but probably indirectly in cats and rats. Eventually, VOR relay neurons mediate the OKR. Thus, the VOR and OKR share the same vestibular relay neurons and act conjointly to stabilize retinal images during head movement. During the OKR, motion is indistinguishable from that induced by head rotation. When eye movements induced by the VOR and OKR exceed certain limits, they are intercalated by quick movements to set back eye position. These oscillatory eye movements are called vestibular or optokinetic nystagmus.

Two other reflexes that act in concert with the VOR and OKR toward the stabilization of retinal images are the cervico-ocular reflex driven by neck torsion and the trunk-ocular reflex elicited by twisting of the trunk. The cervico-ocular reflex is also mediated by the VOR relay neurons; the trunk-ocular reflex may well be mediated by the VOR relay neurons, but this has yet to be confirmed. In addition to these reflexes, proprioceptive signals from extraocular muscles participate in ocular reflex mechanisms, though no stretch reflex can be induced in extraocular muscles. Chronic section of the ophthalmic branch of the trigeminal nerve to interrupt the extraocular muscle afferents causes remarkable instability and slow pendular oscillation of eyes in the dark.

The ocular reflex pathways are attached with several accessory circuits. One is provided by internuclear neurons that interconnect the IIIrd and VIth cranial motor nuclei. In cat

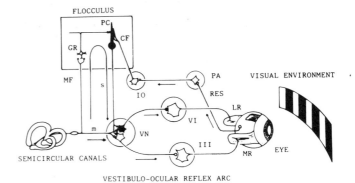

Figure 1. Neuronal connections of the VOR arc and cerebellar flocculus. III and VI, oculomotor and abducens cranial nerve nuclei; VN, vestibular nuclei; LR, lateral rectus muscle; MR, medial rectus muscle; MF, mossy fiber; CF, climbing fiber; PC, Purkinje cell; GR, granule cell; IO, inferior olive; PA, pretectal area; RES, retinal error signal; m, major pathway of the VOR arc; s, floccular pathway to the VOR arc. Inhibitory neurons and synapses are in black, and excitatory ones are left unfilled.

VIth nucleus, about one-third of neurons are internuclear neurons, while the remaining two-thirds are motoneurons. These internuclear neurons receive vestibular inputs similar to abducens motoneurons, and in turn forward excitatory signals to medial rectus motoneurons in the IIIrd nucleus. A corresponding group of internuclear neurons is located in the IIIrd nucleus and adjacent ventral periaqueductal gray matter, and projects to the VIth nucleus region. These internuclear neurons apparently are involved in conjugate activity in the lateral rectus muscle of one eye and the medial rectus muscle of the contralateral eye. Their dysfunction may account for the syndrome of internuclear ophthalmoplegia, a disorder of conjugate lateral gaze.

Another attachment to the ocular reflex pathways is a neural integrator circuit. In the VOR, information about head position is converted to information about eye position. Eye position is represented by the discharge rate of motoneurons for extraocular muscles, while the discharge rate in the primary vestibular nerve fibers generally represents the head angular velocity. Therefore, an integration must be performed in the central pathway for the VOR to convert head velocity signals to head position signals. The same integrator would also be involved in the OKR to convert retinal slip velocity signals to eye position signals. An integrator mechanism, called velocity storage, has also been postulated to account for the prolonged response time constant of VOR relay neurons as compared with the response time constant in the vestibular nerve. The velocity storage produces sustained activity in the oculomotor system outlasting vestibular or optokinetic stimuli, and so accounts for postrotatory nystagmus or oktokinetic afternystagmus. Neural integrator and velocity storage may represent functions of the same neural circuitry, but their identity has yet to be clarified.

A third attachment to ocular reflex pathways is the cerebellum. The cerebellar flocculus receives vestibular afferent signals as a mossy fiber input, and in turn sends Purkinje cell efferent signals to relay cells of the VOR, thus forming a pathway to the VOR arc (Fig. 1). The flocculus also receives visual signals as climbing fiber input. Hence, it has been hypothesized that the floccular pathway to the VOR arc alters its signal transfer characteristics by referring to retinal error signals conveyed by climbing fiber pathways. In other words, the flocculus modifies the overall performance of the VOR to minimize retinal errors and acts as a center of adaptive VOR control. Adaptive VOR control is represented by progressive changes of the VOR gain (ratio of eye movement to head movement) under mismatching of the visual and vestibular environments. For example, wearing dove prism goggles reverses the right-left relationship of the visual field and leads to reduction of VOR gain, and even to reversal of VOR polarity, whereas wearing 2X telescopic lenses leads to increased VOR gain. Sustained rotation of the whole body in combination with the surrounding screen, which represents visual environments, causes similar adaptive changes of VOR gain. In-phase rotation of the whole body and screen leads to a decrease, and out-phase rotation to an increase, of VOR gain.

In accordance with the flocculus hypothesis, VOR adaptability is abolished by lesions of the flocculus or severance of the visual climbing fiber pathway to the flocculus, and discharge patterns of floccular Purkinje cells alter in parallel with VOR gain changes. It has also been demonstrated that responsiveness of floccular Purkinje cells to vestibular mossy fiber inputs can be altered by conjunctive activation of vestibular mossy fibers with climbing fibers, and that the site of this modification is the junction formed on Purkinje cell dendrites by axons of granule cells mediating mossy fiber signals.

Saccade

A saccade is a quick jerky eye movement that positions a visual target on a region of the retina specialized for high acuity. It is essentially voluntary. If a monkey makes a saccade by shifting the direction of gaze from a fixation point to a newly appearing target point, and if the fixation point is extinguished at the same time that the new target appears, the saccadic reaction times are about 200 msec. If the fixation point disappears 15–250 msec before the new target appears, monkeys make regular saccades after shorter reaction times of about 140 msec. In addition, in this gap situation, monkeys make express saccades that have reaction times of no more than 70–80 msec measured from the onset of the new target.

A saccade is generated by a brain stem circuit located in the paramedian zone of the pontine reticular formation (PPRF), which covers the medial portion of the nucleus reticularis magnocellularis between the IVth and VIth nuclei. The PPRF contains several types of neurons that discharge with characteristic response patterns during saccades. Excitatory and inhibitory burst neurons emit characteristic high-frequency (up to 1,000 impulses/sec) bursts, and thereby produce contraction of an eye muscle and relaxation of its antagonist muscle, respectively, during saccades. The second type of saccade-related neurons are pause neurons that stop firing with quick eye movements to one or both sides or with quick eye movements in all directions (omnipause neurons). Omnipause neurons exert monosynaptic inhibitory action on both the excitatory and inhibitory burst neurons and prevent the occurrence of saccades; they should be inhibited for initiation of a saccade. A third group of brain stem neurons are tonic neurons that discharge steadily during fixation, firing at regular tonic rates that alter linearly with eye position. The brain stem saccade generator comprising these neurons will be put into action by driving input signals to excitatory burst neurons, together with suppressing signals to omnipause neurons, from the superior colliculus or the cerebral cortex.

Observations in lesion experiments and in recording from superior colliculus neurons suggest that the superior colliculus computes the vector of saccades based on information about the site of retinal stimulation as well as eye position. The superior colliculus projects to the PPRF as well as the posterior-medial thalamus. In the latter, some cells discharge in relation to saccadic eye movements, and ablation of this structure causes severe and long-lasting deficits in the accuracy of saccades. The posterior-medial thalamus may contain structures critical in guiding saccades to a visual target.

In the cerebral cortex, both the prefrontal eye field and the posterior eye field are involved in generation of saccades. The prefrontal eye field projects to the PPRF, superior colliculus, and pretectal area, where prefrontal cortical signals may intervene in brain stem saccade generator mechanisms. Some prefrontal cortical neurons respond to visual stimuli only when the animal makes a saccade to the stimuli. It is probable that, given a presaccadic enhancement through attention mechanisms, these visually responsive cells in the prefrontal eye field provide retinal error signals to the brain stem saccade generator. Visual responsiveness of posterior eye field neurons also depends on the animals' attention, being enhanced when a light stimulus is the target for saccadic eye movements. A role of posterior eye field saccade neurons may be to facilitate saccade-related processes in the superior colliculus.

Lobules VI and VII of the cerebellum are closely involved in regulation of saccades. Ablation of these cerebellar areas leads to dysmetria in saccades and to inability to adapt to disturbances such as those induced by partial tenotomy in eye muscles. Exact connections of cerebellar lobules VI and VII to the brain stem saccade generater and related higher centers are not known, but it is probable that the cerebellum forms modifiable pathways to the saccade-generating extracerebellar circuitry so as to afford saccade mechanisms with adaptability.

Smooth pursuit

Smooth pursuit is a voluntary movement of eyes which continuously follows a moving target with a high-acuity retinal region. Unlike the OKR, a small dot is an effective target for smooth pursuit movements. For a target moving with a linear constant velocity, the human eye accelerates from rest to any velocity from 5° to 20°/sec in about 130 msec and then follows smoothly. For a sinusoidally moving target, smooth pursuit eye movements follow the target up to 1 Hz, but at higher frequencies pursuit becomes inefficient.

As smooth pursuit eye movement is voluntary, the central command for this movement arises from the cerebral cortex. Some cells were found in the prefrontal eye field in association with smooth pursuit eye movement. Cells in parietal association cortex also respond in relation to smooth pursuit eye movements. It is not clear, however, how the cortical command signals for smooth pursuit are forwarded to the oculomotor system. The cerebellum is also involved in control of smooth pursuit eye movement. Impairment of smooth pursuit and an inability to maintain eccentric gaze occur after himicerebellectomy of monkeys. The deficit is unilateral; the monkey is unable to track with smooth pursuit movements a target moving away from the midline toward the side of the lesion. A lesion localized to the flocculus reduces the gain of the smooth pursuit, but this deficit is less than that induced by total cerebellectomy, suggesting that cerebellar areas other than the flocculus also participate in smooth pursuit eye movements.

Further reading

Symposia
Fuchs AF, Becker W, ed (1981): *Progress in Oculomotor Research.* Amsterdam: Elsevier

Monograph
Carpenter RHS (1977): *Movements of the Eye.* London: Pion
Ito M (1984): *The Cerebellum and Neural Control.* New York: Raven Press

Review article
Fuchs AF, Kaneko CRS (1981): A brain stem generator for saccadic eye movements. *Trend Neurosci* 4:283–286

Optic Nerves, Optic Chiasm, and Optic Tracts

Christopher Walsh

The vertebrate optic nerves, optic chiasm, and optic tracts contain axons of retinal ganglion cells. These axons connect the retina, where light absorption produces patterned neuronal firing, to the brain, where these firing patterns can undergo further processing. The axons are carried in the optic nerve to the optic chiasm at the base of the brain. Beyond the chiasm the axons continue through the optic tract to reach several visual relay nuclei in the brain.

The optic nerve connects two regions of the central nervous system, since the retina and brain both derive from the neural tube. The retina arises as an outpocketing of the neural tube called the optic cup, which remains connected to the immature brain by the optic stalk. The axons of immature retinal ganglion cells then grow out from the optic cup and through the optic stalk to reach the brain. In this way, the stalk fills with fibers to form the optic nerve in the adult.

Projection of retinal fibers in the brain

Axons from the two optic nerves intermingle in the optic chiasm, and then are sorted into the two optic tracts. In each species, the distribution of fibers from one optic nerve into the two optic tracts relates in general to the amount of binocular vision. Thus, in fish the eyes are placed far laterally, and there is little or no binocular vision. The two optic nerves cross one another, with all fibers from each eye going into the opposite optic tract. In animals (such as mammals) in which the eyes are set further forward in the head to allow greater binocular vision, more optic nerve fibers enter the optic tract on the same side of the brain. This partial crossing of retinal fibers is necessary for stereoscopic vision, since it permits fusion in the brain of corresponding retinal images from the two eyes. From such optical considerations Newton correctly deduced the approximate organization of the mammalian optic chiasm long before it could be demonstrated anatomically (see Fig. 1).

The retinal axons project to several relay nuclei in the brain, and each of these projections is precisely organized. In all vertebrates, the retina projects to the optic tectum or its mammalian homolog, the superior colliculus. In mammals, projections to the thalamus, especially the lateral geniculate nucleus, are more highly developed. Further, all animals show several smaller retinal projections. Within each projection, adjacent retinal regions connect to adjacent regions in the brain, producing a straightforward map of the retina (and, hence, of the visual field) among the retinal axon terminals. In animals with binocular vision, inputs from two hemiretinas which view the same part of the visual field (i.e., the nasal, or medial, portion of one retina and the temporal, or lateral, portion of the other) form maps that are exactly aligned with each other (see Fig. 1).

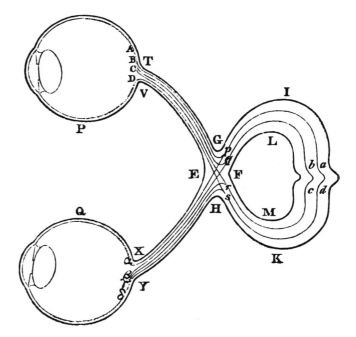

Figure 1. Newton's drawing of the visual pathways. This drawing summarizes schematically several important features of the mammalian visual system. This scheme was deduced by Sir Isaac Newton, based on the necessity for a fusion in the brain of the two binocular images, in order to permit stereoscopic vision. The drawing shows the eyes and the optic nerves, which meet at the optic chiasm. From the chiasm, retinal fibers continue to the brain via the optic tracts. The retinal fibers undergo a partial decussation at the chiasm, with each retina sending part of its input to each side of the brain. Fibers from nasal retina (A,B) cross at the chiasm, and fibers from temporal retina (C,D) project to the same side of the brain. The line of decussation in the retina, which separates cells with crossed axons from cells with uncrossed axons, lies temporal to the optic nerve, between B and C on the right and between β and γ on the left. Each point in the binocular visual field is viewed by corresponding regions in the nasal retina of one eye (α) and the temporal retina of the other (A), and these two images are projected to the same region of the brain (a). The retinal input to the brain is mapped, with adjacent retinal zones (A,B) projecting to adjacent zones in the brain (a,b). This figure also suggests that a similar mapping is present in the optic nerve and tract, but this has not been confirmed anatomically. In other vertebrates with more laterally placed eyes (e.g., fish and frogs) there is less binocular vision, and fewer retinal ganglion cells have uncrossed axons. Some birds, on the other hand, have a high degree of binocular vision, but have a complete crossing of retinal fibers at the optic chiasm. These animals show a functionally equivalent partial crossing of visual fibers at higher levels within the brain. Figure reproduced from Brewster D (1855): *Memoirs of the Life, Writings, and Discoveries of Sir Isaac Newton*, Vol 1, p 433. Edinburgh: Thomas Constable and Co.

The retinal ganglion cells can be subdivided into classes in terms of their size, shape, and functional properties. In the cat, where these cell classes have been studied in detail, each cell class shows its own distinct pattern of projection to the brain. These several ganglion cell types seem to behave as "parallel visual channels," relaying information about different aspects of the visual world (e.g., movement, outlines, color) and forming separate maps in the brain.

Fiber order in the optic nerve

The degree to which these precise retinal mappings seen at terminal locations in the brain also exist in the optic nerve and tract has been the focus of much current research. The earliest descriptions of fiber order in the visual pathway were developed by clinical neurologists who found blind spots for localized portions of the visual field in association with fairly distinct lesions of the human optic nerve or optic tract discovered at autopsy. They reasoned that these lesions in the pathway must have killed axons from a small spot on the retina, and concluded that the optic nerve contained a simple map of the retina, while the optic tract contained two overlapping, precisely aligned maps of the two corresponding hemiretinas, similar to the maps formed in the brain by axon terminals.

This traditional view, while possibly true in humans, has been called into question by recent studies in experimental animals. In the cat's optic nerve, fibers from adjacent ganglion cells take widely divergent routes. Further, electron microscopic analysis of the fetal monkey's optic nerve shows that growing retinal axons become widely separated from their neighbors. Thus, any retinal mapping that may exist in the nerve near the eye is lost nearer the brain, although the rules for these fiber rearrangements are not known.

The rules governing fiber ordering in the optic nerve of several nonmammalian vertebrates have been worked out in greater detail. These animals add new ganglion cells to the retina as concentric rings, and age-related retinal fibers are generally grouped together in the nerve. Other features of fiber ordering differ among species. For example, the chick's retina is represented in the nerve as if it were folded in half along its vertical midline, and in the frog the retinal representation is duplicated along the vertical midline. The fiber patterns in the nerve can also undergo substantial rearrangements along its length. While these reorganizations usually preserve the grouping of axons by age, the mapping of the retina is often obscured.

Common principles of fiber order in the optic tract

Despite the variety of fiber patterns seen in the optic nerve, the optic tract shows similar rules of fiber organization in all vertebrates. Again, the key to this fiber ordering is relative age, with the oldest fibers being the deepest in the tract, and newer fibers nearer the surface of the tract. In nonmammalian vertebrates, retinal axons from the concentric, age-related retinal rings are arranged as layers parallel to the surface of the tract. This fiber order reflects the sequence of axon ingrowth, with fibers from each new age-related ring entering the tract in an orderly manner along its outer margin, displacing older fibers to deeper levels in the tract.

The same general rules apply to fiber order in the mammalian optic tract, with the cat being the mammal most closely studied. At first sight the fiber arrangement in the cat's optic tract looks extremely complex, since axons of the different ganglion cell size classes are partially segregated into different zones of the tract. In fact, each of these ganglion cell size classes seems to form a separate retinal map in the tract, resulting in several rough, overlapping maps in the tract that are out of alignment with one another.

These several maps also represent the sequence of arrival of retinal axons in the optic tract during development, with the newest axons along the surface of the tract. However, this relationship is less obvious than in frogs and fish, because retinal development in mammals does not occur by a simple addition of concentric rings of cells. Instead, the several ganglion cell size classes are added as several separate, partially overlapping waves of cell production, each wave starting near the central retina and spreading gradually toward the periphery. This chronological sequence of ganglion cell addition corresponds to the spatial relationships established by the retinal axons in the tract.

Although in all vertebrates the optic tract shows a grouping of fibers by age, topographic maps of the retina formed in the tract differ somewhat. While in frogs and fish the fibers from the four retinal quadrants are segregated, in the chick's optic tract, as in the chick's optic nerve, the retina is represented as folded along the vertical midline, with overlapping maps of the nasal and temporal hemiretinas from one eye. In the cat, although maps from nasal and temporal hemiretinas overlap, these maps receive input from the nasal retina of one eye and the temporal retina of the other eye. In all cases, the optic tract order can be viewed as a rough presorting of the retinal axons in terms of their connections in the brain, with axons deeper in the tract terminating in general deeper in the brain. However, the terminal mapping is always far more precise than the fiber mapping, and thus the former is not explicable merely in terms of the latter.

Fiber growth and fiber order

The differing patterns of fiber order in the optic nerve and optic tract seem to reflect changing cellular relationships along the route from eye to brain. In the fetal optic nerve, the retinal axons are embedded among glial cells that wrap the axons to form bundles. The morphological relationships of the optic stalk change rapidly with age and vary widely among species. In contrast, the optic tract develops at the surface of the brain, with growing axons always relating to the outer processes of structurally uniform, radially oriented neuroepithelial cells. The axons add in layers just beneath the surface, and there are no axon bundles. This surface addition, which naturally produces a grouping of fibers by age, may be quite common throughout the nervous system of all vertebrates. However, surface addition cannot explain all aspects of retinal fiber growth, since axons leave the surface where they make synaptic contacts. Furthermore, surface addition cannot explain the orderly, separate mapping of the retinal quadrants (in the tract and in the brain), nor can it explain the species differences in the mapping of the quadrants in the tract. These other aspects of fiber growth presumably depend on other cellular mechanisms not yet well understood. Although Newton could deduce much about the adult structure of the visual system without knowledge of the cells which make it up, much remains to be learned about how this visual structure is realized through cellular interactions during neural development.

Acknowledgements

Supported by NIH grant 5T32 GM-07281.

Further reading

Guillery RW (1983): The optic chiasm of the vertebrate brain. In: *Contributions to Sensory Physiology*, Vol 7, Neff WD, ed. New York: Academic Press

Miller NR (1984): *Walsh and Hoyt's Clinical Neuro-ophthalmology*, Vol 1, 4th ed. Baltimore: Williams and Wilkins

Polyak S (1957): *The Vertebrate Visual System*, Klüver H, ed. Chicago: University of Chicago Press

Optic Tectum

David J. Ingle

In nonmammalian vertebrates the optic tectum is the largest and most conspicuous visual center: its twin lobes are literally the roof of the midbrain, as implied by its Latin root. Each tectal lobe receives the majority of retinal fibers from the contralateral eye, and these are distributed in a precise retinotopic order such that contralateral visual space is mapped out on the surface of the tectum. The great convenience of defining this mapping order by means of microelectrode recordings or by various anatomical tracer methods has made the tecta of amphibians and fish popular structures for developmental and regeneration studies aimed at elucidating the underlying mechanisms for guidance of retinal axons toward their cellular targets in the brain. The tectal motor map is activated by retinal input and descends via efferent pathways to brain stem and spinal motor centers. This has been demonstrated in a few species (trout, cod, toad, and alligator) by electrically stimulating the various regions of optic tectum in a freely behaving animal. Activation of rostral tectum elicits short turns of head or body toward the frontal field; stimulation of caudal tectum elicits large orientations designed to fixate stimuli appearing contralaterally in the rear field. Although the optic tectum resembles its mammalian homolog, the superior colliculus, it differs in that most of its descending efferent neurons are in direct contact with incoming retinal fibers. Three key questions under current investigation are these: (1) What kinds of afferent input trigger orienting behavior? (2) Which efferent pathways mediate specific response components? (3) How is the input-output transformation facilitated or inhibited by other nonretinal inputs to tectum?

Feeding behavior

In fishes and frogs direct electrical-point stimulation can elicit either turn-to-fixate movements or a lunge-and-snap at rostral stimuli. Film analysis of frogs reveals that along a given line of sight the animal may either snap at or merely fixate a prey stimulus, depending upon its distance from the eye. Therefore, in most regions of the frog's tectum there must be output neurons that can activate either the localizing or the consummatory response (see Fig. 1). Studies show that severing the contralateral efferent tectal projection (by splitting the ventral tegmentum where these fibers cross) will eliminate turning toward prey, while the animal retains the ability to jump and snap forward to stimuli anywhere in the visual field. An opposite deficit can be induced by a hemisection of the brain just caudal to tectum, eliminating descending ipsilateral fibers. Such frogs can turn and fixate more distant stimuli, but cannot snap at nearby prey in the lateral visual fields. Backfilling ipsilateral or contralateral efferent channels with horseradish peroxidase reveals that the tectal cells of origin of the two systems have distinctive dendritic morphology and presumably receive different patterns of visual input. Details of synaptic

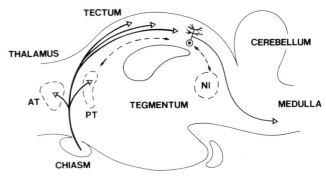

Figure 1. A schematic view of the frog's optic tectum in a midsagittal section. The best studied afferent and efferent pathways are emphasized. The dark lines with arrows represent the main excitatory input from the eye, via the optic tract, which ascends from the optic chiasm and enters the tectum in three distinct sublaminae, the long efferent axons from tectum that reach the brain stem and spinal cord. The dashed lines show two-way connections between tectum, on one hand, and two other well-studied visual centers: the pretectal region (PT) rostrally and the nucleus isthmi (NI) caudally. The two sets of interconnections may include circuits for feedback modulation of intrinsic tectal neurons. Not shown are inputs from telencephalon and tegmentum, two-way connections with the anterior thalamus (AT), and direct intertectal projections.

contacts between afferent fibers and these identified efferent neurons are likely to be worked out by newly developed methods of electron microscopy that label both neural elements.

The retinal inputs to tecta of several groups have already been examined in some detail by single-unit recording methods. J. Y. Lettvin and colleagues were the first to demonstrate in the frog that distinctive functional types of ganglion cell axons (e.g., moving-spot detectors, on-off units, and dark detectors) terminate at different layers below the tectal surface. Although fish, reptilian, and avian tecta are similarly laminated histologically, the same degree of laminar segregation of various optic fiber types (motion detectors, color sensors, on-off units) has not been demonstrated. For the frog it appears likely that moving-spot detectors provide a key input for triggering the fixation response to moving insects, while snapping at nearby (large angle) stimuli appears also to be triggered by off-on units. Since fishes, reptiles, and birds typically show turning-fixating responses to food stimuli, it seems likely that a similar retinal-tectal circuitry mediates these exploratory and feeding behaviors. It must be noted that birds and reptiles frequently display a head-cocking response to novel stimuli that brings the visual image to a central fovea, in addition to fixating objects via a binocular region of retina preparatory to striking or pecking forward. Thus the output channels from tectum in birds and reptiles may be more complicated.

Avoidance behavior

Both frogs and fishes typically respond to looming dark objects by flipping or jumping away in the opposite direction. The dark detectors found in the tectum of both groups probably contribute to this reflexive escape behavior. In both groups, removal of tectum abolishes this visually elicited escape response as well as eliminating visually induced feeding. This system probably exhibits more complexity than a simple sensitivity to increasing darkness, since frogs discriminate at a distance stimuli approaching on a collision course from those that will narrowly miss them. Avoidance behavior is also well integrated with localization of obstacles (which are avoided) and detection of distant dark areas (which are approached as holes for hiding). Thus, the avoidance movement sequences elicited by threat are determined by activity in other visual centers.

Nonretinal inputs

A major source of modulating input to the tectum is the pretectal region of the caudal thalamus. Fibers from two large pretectal cell groups (lateral and posterior groups) terminate at different levels of the ipsilateral tectum (Fig. 1). Large lesions of pretectum (or even focal lesions of the lateral nucleus) appear to release the tectum from tonic inhibition, as seen by the excessive feeding behavior of frogs and toads with pretectal damage. These animals lose the normal size selectivity of prey catching and will strike at very large objects that they normally avoid. Furthermore, the habituation of feeding to continually moving dummy stimuli is abolished by pretectum ablation. These effects have their correlates in responsiveness of certain intrinsic tectal cells. Lesions of pretectum in the toad will abolish the selectivity of certain cells for narrow wormlike objects and render them excitable by large squares. Habituation properties of a similar class of cells in the frog's tectum were abolished as well after pretectal lesions. Since pretectal connections to tectum are prominent in all vertebrates, it seems likely that further investigation of other vertebrate groups will reveal an analogous modulatory role of this diencephalic area upon tectum.

Another important source of input to the tectum is from a satellite system, the nucleus isthmus, which is homologous to the parabigeminal nucleus in mammals. In frogs (and also in mammals), this system receives a highly retinotopic projection from the ipsilateral tectum and sends fibers to both the ipsilateral and contralateral tecta (Fig. 1). In fishes, reptiles, and birds, a similar structure receives tectal input but sends return axons only to the ipsilateral tectum. The frog has a wide binocular visual field, and indeed one can easily record a prominent ipsilateral visual projection on the rostral (binocular) zone of the tectum. This projection disappears when the contralateral nucleus isthmus is lesioned or when the crossing fibers in the postoptic commissure are cut. The exact function of this isthmus relay is unknown, since destruction of the isthmi is reported to spare the use of binocular disparity cues for estimation of prey-striking distance by toads. However, some tectal units on the ipsilateral and contralateral side appear to be disinhibited acutely following isthmic lesions, so that future studies of this large input system should be rewarding.

Several lower vertebrate species have in common with their mammalian cousins the existence of prominent multimodal inputs to the tectum. For example, tectal neurons of electric gymnotid fish respond to motion of a dielectric object within the near lateral space, the excitation being relayed to tectum from the electrosensory afferent system. Some units will respond to both visual and electrosensory events in the same location. Tectal units of congenitally blind cave fish are sensitive to movement of objects in contralateral space, relayed via the lateral line system of the VIIIth cranial nerve. This is likely to be true for some sighted fish as well. An analogous arrangement is seen in the pit viper where some deep tectal neurons are excited (or inhibited) by a localized heat source in front of the snake, detected by the heat-focusing pit organs of the snout and relayed to the brain by a branch of the trigeminal nerve. A variety of interactions between heat localization inputs and visual inputs have been documented in this snake, although the significance of such interactions for behavior is still speculative. In these and other instances of intermodal convergence in the tectum, it is not known whether nonvisual inputs only modulate responsiveness to visual targets or whether they substitute for vision and directly elicit orienting or striking behavior.

Other inputs to the tectum include those from large cells of the tegmentum (which have been compared with the mammalian nigrotectal system) and descending projections from regions of the telencephalon. Both sets of inputs provide putative routes for modulation of feeding or avoidance tendencies by motivational systems and for modification of behavior by conditioning. Initial reports that telencephalic inputs to tectum are lacking in frogs appear to have been contradicted by more sensitive methods using tracers such as horseradish peroxidase. However, the loci of telencephalofugal projections to the tectum appear to vary within each vertebrate class or order. Comparative behavioral studies of factors influencing those feeding and avoidance behaviors mediated by the tectum should therefore provide insight into the functional organization of the telencephalon itself.

Further reading

Ewert JP (1974): The neural basis of visually guided behavior. *Sci Am* 230:34–42

Ingle D (1973): Two visual systems in the frog. *Science* 181:1053–1055

Ingle D (1983): Brain mechanisms of localization in frogs and toads. In: *Advances in Vertebrate Neuroethology*, Ewert JP, Capranica RR, Ingle DJ, eds. New York: Plenum

Vanegas H (ed) (1984): *Comparative Neurology of the Optic Tectum*. New York: Plenum

Reading

Marcel Kinsbourne

The skill of reading is uniquely placed in brain research. It is the most widely practiced skill that humans specifically learn (in contrast to spoken speech, which is acquired without deliberate instruction). As such it offers opportunities for research on the brain representation of cognitive skills. (Are they modular, incorporating a single "reading center," or componential, using multiple component processes diversely localized?) Because of its great practical importance and the wide range of individual difference in its acquisition and ultimate level of performance, investigators have attempted to determine the nature of reading mechanisms, their brain basis, and the nature of the differences between skilled and unskilled readers (quantitative or qualitative). Particular attention is currently paid to the question of why dyslexics experience disproportionate difficulty in learning to read for reasons of brain maturation (rather than environmental deficiency).

The vast bulk of reading research is centered on the Western alphabetic script. Ideographic and syllabic scripts used in the Orient have also been studied to provide a counterpoint to Western reading research.

People learn to read through pattern analysis (whole-word approach), phonics analysis (the establishment of grapheme-phoneme correspondences), and phonological and linguistic analysis with such regularities as exist in the language. The choice of method presumably depends on the language used, as some (e.g., German, Spanish, and Italian) exhibit far more regular grapheme-phoneme correspondence than others (e.g., English and the Scandinavian languages). However, although emphasis differs among teachers and across generations as styles change, it is generally hard to find out which method a child has been taught by (except perhaps in individualized remedial settings). Although the way they have been taught should affect the type of difficulties children encounter at various levels of reading acquisition and could be relevant to learning blocks, the fitting of remedial methodology to the individual is based on clinical opinion.

Reading instruction generally begins between ages 5 and 7 in a classroom. There is reason to suppose that most children could be taught a significant degree of reading skill much earlier on an individualized and noncompetitive basis. Whether this is desirable is disputed: Opponents wish to shield children from competitive pressures: advocates stress the advantage to a child of acquiring an easy familiarity with the reading process before being placed in a more formal group situation.

Most experts accept the concept of reading readiness, that is, minimal competence in relevant cognitive processes that a child needs before he can profit from reading instruction. The concept is weakened, however, by our ignorance as to what these component processes might be and how they might be measured independent of the actual reading activity. Although investigators have assumed that a variety of mental operations performed outside reading are sufficiently general to be involved in reading itself, there is no proof of this. Screening tests for reading readiness have generally proved insufficiently predictive to be of practical use. When the test clearly predicts a child unready to learn to read, this was already obvious to more casual observation.

Whereas it is clear that many children may achieve reading readiness well before school entry, some apparently do not for years afterward. That fact should not be construed as indicating that they are unteachable. Rather, their learning requirements are individual and, to be met, require individualized methodologies. In other words they have learning disabilities. As this is a problem of major dimensions, many methodologies have been advocated for "remediation" of learning disabilities, but beyond customary individual treatment, there is no systematic evidence that any one of them works better than the others, or even that as a package they work. Because of the dubious success of remedial methods for reading disability and because of the high level of illiteracy and semiliteracy that persists, reading disability has been the target of a major research effort with neuroscience implications. Investigators have attempted to incriminate either structural or functional deficits in the brain of dyslexics. Suggestions have ranged from those of specific neuronal damage or dysgenesis in the left hemispheric language area, through disorders of brain organization (e.g., overlapping representation of verbal and spatial skills in one hemisphere), to insufficient selective activation of relevant cerebral areas. It has further been suggested that reading disability should be subtyped to reflect the selective impairment of different components of the reading process. But none of the currently advocated patterns of subtypes has thoroughly established validity. Nor has any of this effort translated into validated improved remedial methodology.

One potential source of subtyping is by analogy between types of developmental reading disability and syndromes of alexia caused by focal brain damage in people who are already fluent readers. Alexia was one of the earliest concepts introduced by connectionist neuropsychologists. Dating from Déjerine's report in 1892, they conceived of a reading center located in the left posterior cerebrum and separate from the language center, which could be either impaired or disconnected from other centers that would mediate its output. More recent evidence has tended to discredit this approach and substitute an account of syndromes of acquired reading disability in terms of impairment of one or more components essential to the reading process. A major question within this approach has been whether the reader can directly derive meaning from print or has to pass through an intermediary articulatory state, during which he subvocalizes the sounds of the words he sees and therefrom infers the meaning. Evidence from cognitive psychology suggests that fluent reading bypasses such an articulatory stage, and evidence from selective brain damage supports this. A dissociation exists between phonological dyslexics, who can read familiar words, but cannot decode unfamiliar or nonwords, and surface dyslexics, who have lost sight reading skills, but retain the ability to use a phonics approach to decoding. A dissociation also exists between reading for sound and for meaning. Some patients (direct dyslexics) can read words aloud but without any comprehension. Other patients (deep dyslexics) cannot decode print into sound and yet can gather what it means. A persisting problem in any such process is whether the abnormal performance studied represents the best efforts of an impaired reading system to proceed or a qualitatively different alternative approach by undamaged areas (particularly right hemisphere) to substitute for the damaged reading facility on the left.

While most alexic patients are also aphasic and agraphic, the existence of dissociations between these components of language is of theoretical interest. The syndrome of pure alexia (alexia without agraphia), if validated, implies that a topo-graphically distinctive brain area subserves word and even letter identification. However, in those studies in which it has been adequately tested, visual identification of other stimuli (digits, shapes, colors) has also been found impaired. It therefore remains an open question whether a special-purpose module for reading exists in the brain, or whether alexia without agraphia is only the clinically most obtrusive manifestation of a more general deficit in rapid visual identification.

Further reading

Coltheart TM, Patterson K, Marshall JC (1980): *Deep Dyslexia*. London: Routledge and Kegan Paul

Gibson EJ, Levin H (1975): *The Psychology of Reading*. Cambridge: MIT Press

Kinsbourne M, Caplan PJ (1979): *Children's Learning and Attention Problems*. Boston: Little, Brown

Retina, Neurotransmitters

Dianna A. Redburn

The six major classes of retinal neurons (photoreceptor, horizontal, bipolar, amacrine, interplexiform, and ganglion cells) each have several subtypes, providing a grand total of about 60 recognized classes of retinal neurons. The neurotransmitters used by approximately 80% of these functionally distinct populations correspond to one of six different classical neurotransmitters, and/or one of a variety of neuropeptides representing eight different peptide families.

Visual information is initially encoded in rod and cone photoreceptor cells via visual transduction, and subsequently transmitted from photoreceptors to bipolars to ganglion cells through chemical synapses which use an acidic amino acid, probably glutamate. Since light causes hyperpolarization of photoreceptors, the rate of glutamate release from these cells is directly proportional to the degree of tonic, dark-induced depolarization of the photoreceptor terminal and inversely proportional to the amount of photopigment bleached. Glutamate has opposite effects on two classes of cone bipolar cells; it depolarizes one set (OFF bipolars) and hyperpolarizes another (ON bipolars). Thus OFF bipolars are driven by direct glutamate depolarization in the dark, and ON bipolars are driven by disinhibition (loss of glutamate hyperpolarization) in the light. Both ON and OFF bipolars probably release glutamate from their terminals and cause direct excitation of ganglion cells. The single class of rod bipolars have responses similar to that of OFF cone bipolars.

Horizontal cells, as the name implies, produce horizontal integration in the outer plexiform layer among photoreceptor-to-bipolar synapses. They are depolarized by glutamate and at least one subclass utilizes gamma-aminobutyric acid (GABA) as a neurotransmitter. There is some evidence that GABA may be released from horizontal cells by the conventional calcium-dependent, stimulus-coupled-secretion mechanism characteristic of other neurons and in addition through a calcium-independent mechanism that may represent a reversal of the GABA uptake system. GABAergic horizontal cells are both pre- and postsynaptic to photoreceptor cells and provide inhibitory feedback loops that modulate the temporal properties of the photoreceptor response. Since horizontal cells are electrically coupled via gap junctions, they have very broad receptive fields. It is this property that subserves another GABA-related function in the outer plexiform layer, namely, the establishment of center-surround characteristics of bipolar cells and hence other retina neurons. Illumination of the center of a bipolar cell's receptive field produces either an ON or OFF response as a result of direct photoreceptor input. In contrast, illumination of the area surrounding the center produces the opposite response as a result of antagonistic horizontal cell input directly on bipolars or indirectly through photoreceptors.

In addition to glutamatergic input from photoreceptors, horizontal cells also receive dopaminergic input from interplexiform cells. Interplexiform cells form feedback loops with input from the inner plexiform layer and output primarily to the outer plexiform layer. Dopamine released from one class of interplexiform cells activates D1 (adenylate cyclase stimulating) receptors on horizontal cells, and causes a decrease in the conductance of gap junctions among horizontal cells. The receptive field size of the horizontal cell is reduced, thus leading to a modification of the center-surround properties of other retinal neurons. Other classes of interplexiform cells appear to use GABA or glycine as a neurotransmitter but their function is unknown.

Amacrine cells represent a highly diverse cell population containing approximately 25 different subclasses. Most types exhibit highly laminated terminal fields within the inner plexiform layer, where they contact other amacrines as well as bipolar, interplexiform and ganglion cells with reciprocal and serial synapses. Through asymmetries in their terminal fields, GABAergic and glycinergic amacrines provide inhibitory influences that establish size, velocity, orientation, and directionally selective responses in ganglion cells. As many as three different glycinergic and five different GABAergic amacrines play an active role in establishing these complex receptive field characteristics of ganglion cells.

An additional subclass of glycinergic amacrine cell, named AII or A7, is thought to play a unique role in scotopic vision by providing a link between rod bipolar cells and ganglion cells; no direct synaptic connection between these two cells has been observed. The A7 glycinergic cell receives synaptic input from rods and in turn forms electrotonic gap junctions with other A7 cells and with cone bipolars. Thus it appears that scotopic visual information from rod photoreceptors reaches ganglion cells via cone bipolar terminals. The potential for indiscriminate mixing of rod and cone signals within the same cone terminal may be controlled by dopamine from interplexiform or amacrine cells that may modulate conductance of these gap junctions similar to the dopamine regulation of horizontal cell gap junctions. Dopamine represents the major catecholamine transmitter found in retinas of most species. The sparse distribution of norepinephrine and epinephrine terminals found in retinas of some species primarily represents retinal afferents that originate from other brain structures. The pathways described above are summarized in Figure 1.

Serotonin is also utilized as a transmitter by specific subclasses of amacrine cells. Although the functions of these cells are unclear, at least one subclass displays a synaptic pattern similar to that of the glycinergic A7 cell and thus may provide a link in scotopic circuitry.

Acetylcholine (ACh) is the transmitter of starburst amacrine cells, so named because of their extensive and symmetrical terminal array. In addition to glutamate, ACh provides another excitatory input to ganglion cells through nicotinic receptors and thus represents an exception from the general inhibitory

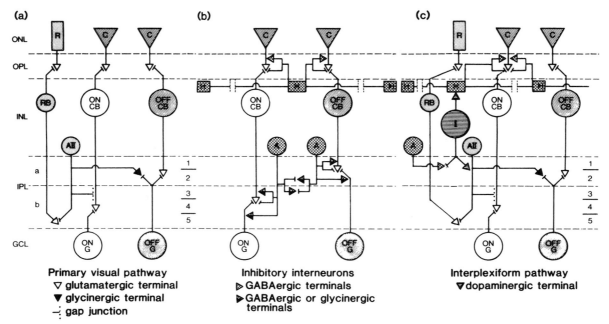

Figure 1. General circuit diagram for the vertebrate retina. a. The primary visual or vertical pathway for cones involves three major cell types, all of which probably use glutamate as a neurotransmitter. Cones have cell bodies (C) in the outer nuclear layer (ONL). In the outer plexiform layer (OPL) they synapse with ON and OFF cone bipolars (CB), which in turn synapse with ON and OFF ganglion cells (G) in sublamina a (layers 1 and 2) and sublamina b (layers 3, 4, and 5), respectively, within the inner plexiform layer (IPL). Elements of the cone pathway that are depolarized during the dark are shaded. Elements that are depolarized by light are not shaded.

The direct pathway for rods also involves three specific cell types (stippled). Rods (R) synapse with rod bipolars (RB), which in turn synapse

with glycinergic amacrine cells (A II, also called A7) in sublamina b. The A II cell synapses on OFF ganglion cells in sublamina a and forms gap junctions with ON bipolar cells. b. Lateral pathways are formed by two major types of interneurons with somas (cross-hatched) in the inner nuclear layer INL. In the outer retina, horizontal cells (H) (some of which are GABAergic) provide negative feedback to photoreceptors and are themselves coupled through gap junctions. In the inner retina, GABAergic and glycinergic amacrine cells form feedback loops with both ON and OFF bipolar cells and they are presynaptic to ganglion cells. c. Amacrine cells also synapse on interplexiform cells (I) which send information back to the OPL through synapses on horizontal cells. GABA and dopamine are the neurotransmitters utilized in at least one such pathway.

nature of most amacrines. Cholinergic terminals are confined to two narrowly stratified laminae in the inner plexiform layer. The outermost band originates from conventionally placed amacrines in the inner nuclear layer, and along with bipolar terminals which are also found in this sublamina, these cells are involved in activity of the OFF circuit. In contrast, the innermost band originates from amacrines whose cell bodies are displaced to the ganglion cell layer, and along with bipolar terminals found within this sublamina, these cells are involved in activity of the ON circuit. Cholinergic amacrines are driven by glutamate input from bipolars or perhaps from a population of poorly understood glutamatergic amacrines, and they are inhibited by glycine and GABA. It has been suggested that GABA may establish the directionally sensitive properties of ganglion cells indirectly via its action on cholinergic amacrines.

Somatostatin, substance P, neuroactive peptide Y, enkephalin, vasoactive intestinal peptide, glucagon, cholecystokinin, thyrotropin-releasing hormone, and neurotensin are examples from the rapidly growing list of peptides whose antibodies show cross-reactivity in retina. Based on immunoreactivity, most neuropeptides appear to be localized within specific subsets of amacrine cells. Some are thought to be co-localized with a classical neurotransmitter, for example, GABA and enkephalin, neurotensin and glycine. Immunohistochemical staining for most retinal neuropeptides reveals a surprisingly uniform, trilaminar pattern located in inner, middle, and outer regions (sublaminae 1, 3, and 5) of the inner plexiform layer. In general peptides may provide slow-acting, long-term modu-

lation of amacrine cell networks; however, important exceptions such as the rapid effects of enkephalins on ganglion cells are already apparent.

Like their counterparts the pinealocytes, retinal photoreceptors synthesize and release both serotonin and melatonin. As in the pineal, retinal synthesis of melatonin is stimulated by darkness via a cAMP cascade involving the rate-limiting, synthetic enzyme, n-acetyl transferase. Melatonin diffuses freely from the cell so that the appearance of extracellular melatonin is regulated primarily via its synthesis rather than stimulus-coupled secretion mechanisms characteristic of neurotransmitters. The role of melatonin in retinal function is still speculative but hormone-like effects on photoreceptor outer segments and pigment epithelium have been noted.

Further reading

Dowling JE, Dubin MW (1982): *The Vertebrate Retina*. In: *Handbook of Physiology*, Vol 2, Greiger SR, ed. Baltimore: American Physiological Society

Kolb H, Nelson R (1984): Neural architecture of the cat retina. In: *Progress in Retinal Research*, Vol 3, Osborne NN, Chader GJ, eds. Oxford: Pergamon Press

Massey SC, Redburn DA (1986): Transmitter circuits in the vertebrate retina. In: *Progress in Neurobiology*, Phillis JW, ed. New York: Pergamon Press, in press

Miller RF, Slaughter RF (1985): Excitatory amino acid receptors in the vertebrate retina. In: *Retinal Transmitters and Modulators: Models for the Brain*, Vol 2, Morgan WW, ed. Boca Raton: CRC Press

Retina, Vertebrate

John E. Dowling

The vertebrate retina, lining the pigment epithelium along the back of the eye, is a part of the central nervous system and in all species is constructed according to the same basic plan (Fig. 1).

Two synaptic layers, the outer and inner plexiform layers, are interspersed between three cellular layers, the outer and inner nuclear and ganglion cell layers. Light, entering the eye, passes through the transparent retina and is captured by the most distal retinal elements, the photoreceptors (rods and cones) whose cell perikarya make up the outer nuclear layer. The inner nuclear layer contains the perikarya of four types of neurons, the horizontal, bipolar, amacrine, and interplexiform cells, while the most proximal cellular layer contains the perikarya of the third-order ganglion cells. Exceptions to this organization are that horizontal and bipolar cells can occasionally be found in the outer nuclear layer, ganglion cells in the inner nuclear layer, and amacrine cells in the ganglion cell layer. The major glial elements in the retina, the Müller cells, extend vertically through the retinal thickness; their nuclei are usually found in the inner nuclear layer.

Almost all synapses in the retina are confined to the two plexiform layers and in each of these two layers, the processes of four cell types interact. In the outer plexiform layer are found processes of the photoreceptor, horizontal, bipolar, and interplexiform cells while in the inner plexiform layer are found the processes of bipolar, amacrine, ganglion, and interplexiform cells. The photoreceptors provide the input to the outer plexiform layer, while the bipolar cells are the output neurons for that synaptic layer. Input to the inner plexiform layer is provided by the bipolar terminals while the output neurons of that layer, and indeed the entire retina, are the ganglion cells whose axons form the optic nerve. The processes of horizontal and amacrine cells are usually confined to the outer plexiform or inner plexiform layers respectively, while the interplexiform cells appear to be primarily centrifugal neurons, carrying information from inner to outer plexiform layer, and spreading processes in both layers.

Functional organization

Electron microscopic studies have provided information concerning the synaptic organization of the retina. For example, in the outer plexiform layer, receptors synapse onto bipolar cell dendrites and horizontal cell processes while in several species, horizontal cell synapses are observed on bipolar cell dendrites. Thus receptors appear to drive both the bipolar and horizontal cells, whereas horizontal cells provide a pathway for lateral interactions between distant receptors and bipolar cells.

In the inner plexiform layer, bipolar cell terminals synaptically contact ganglion cell dendrites and amacrine cell processes. Amacrine cell processes make feedback synapses on

bipolar terminals, feedforward synapses on ganglion cell dendrites, and lateral synapses on other amacrine processes. Classes of ganglion cells that differ in terms of type of synaptic input are indicated from electron microscopic studies of Golgi-impregnated cells. Some ganglion cells receive substantial input from bipolar cell terminals, and others receive their input primarily, if not exclusively, from amacrine cell processes.

Intracellular recordings from the retinal neurons extend the understanding of retinal synaptic organization (Fig. 2). Distal retinal neurons (receptor, horizontal, and bipolar cells) respond to light with sustained, graded potentials. Receptors hyperpolarize in response to illumination of a limited retinal area, while horizontal cells hyperpolarize to illumination over a much wider area. Bipolar cells of two types have been described: one responds by depolarizing to centered-spot illumination; the other, by hyperpolarizing to centered-spot illumination. Figure 2 shows only responses of a center-hyperpolarizing bipolar cell. Surround illumination in both bipolar cell types produces a response that is opposite in polarity to the response of central illumination. The center response of bipolar cells appears to be mediated by direct receptor-bipolar cell interaction, whereas the surround response is provided by an antagonistic horizontal cell input feeding forward onto the bipolar cell dendrites or back onto receptor terminals. The horizontal cells have a wider process spread than bipolar cells, and thus an antagonistic center-surround organization is established in the bipolar cells and in some receptors.

In the inner plexiform layer many amacrine cells depolarize transiently at the on and off of illumination, and others respond with sustained depolarizing or hyperpolarizing responses. Figure 2 shows only a transient type of amacrine cell response. Amacrine cells may generate action potentials, as do all ganglion cells. Ganglion cells of two basic classes are encountered in many retinas. One class responds more or less tonically to illumination, giving an on or an off response to centered-spot illumination. The receptive field of this class of ganglion cell shows a center-surround antagonistic organization like that of the bipolar cells described above. The second class of ganglion cell responds transiently at the on and off of illumination and usually responds vigorously to moving stimuli and often to directional stimuli. It has been proposed that the ganglion cells showing the more sustained responses and the center-surround receptive field organization receive their input primarily from bipolar cells and sustained amacrine cells, whereas the ganglion cells showing transient activity and motion sensitivity receive their input primarily from the transient amacrine cell system.

As noted above, interplexiform cells appear to be centrifugal neurons. They receive all their input in the inner plexiform layer from amacrine cells, and while they make some synapses onto amacrine cells, most of their output is in the outer plexiform layer on horizontal and/or bipolar cells. In fish, these

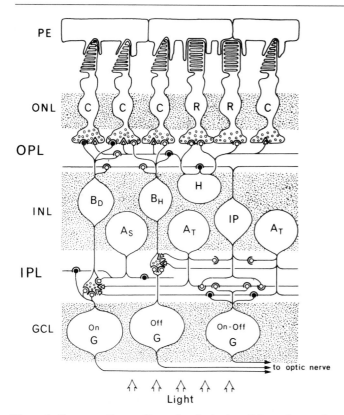

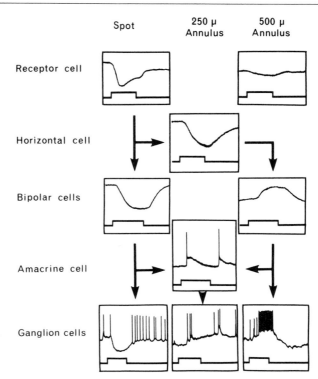

Figure 1. Summary diagram illustrating the basic cellular and synaptic organization of the vertebrate retina. Two synaptic layers, the outer and inner plexiform layers (OPL and IPL) are interspersed between three cellular layers, the outer and inner nuclear layers and ganglion cell layers (ONL, INL, and GCL). The cell bodies (perikarya) of the cone and rod photoreceptors (C and R) make up the ONL; horizontal (H), bipolar (B), amacrine (A), and interplexiform (IP) cell perikarya make up the INL. Ganglion cell perikarya, (G) make up the GCL. Excitatory synapses (open circles) inhibitory synapses (closed circles), and reciprocal synapses (triangles) are indicated in each plexiform layer. Two types of bipolar cells are indicated, those that depolarize in response to spot illumination (B_D), and those that hyperpolarize to spot illumination (B_H). Because depolarizing bipolars terminate in the lower half of the IPL, most on-responses are generated in that part of the IPL. Conversely, most off-responses are generated in the upper part of the IPL where the hyperpolarizing bipolars terminate. Two types of amacrine cells are also indicated, those that respond to light with sustained potentials (A_S) and those that respond with transient potentials (A_T). Through the synaptic interactions occurring in each synaptic layer, the receptive field properties of the on- and off-center ganglion cells and on-off ganglion cells are formed.

Figure 2. Intracellular responses from receptor, horizontal, bipolar, amacrine, and ganglion cells of the mudpuppy retina. The distal retinal neurons (receptor, horizontal, and bipolar cells) respond to illumination with graded sustained potentials; the proximal retinal neurons show both sustained and transient potentials and action potentials. The receptor, bipolar, and ganglion cells respond differently to center (spot) and surround (annular) illumination. Horizontal and amacrine cells usually respond similarly to spot and annular illumination; here responses to a small annulus (250 μm) are shown which stimulates both the center and surround of the receptive field. The bipolar cell illustrated is a center-hyperpolarizing cell, the amacrine cell shown is a transient amacrine cell, and the ganglion cell is an off-center cell. The arrows indicate in a general way how the responses are synaptically generated. That is, the receptor cells directly drive the horizontal and bipolar cells. Bipolar cell responses evoked with a large annulus (right side) are generated by horizontal cell activity. The bipolar cells provide the major input for amacrine cell responses and the responses of the off- and on-center ganglion cells. The transient amacrine cells provide the major input for the on-off ganglion cells (center record).

neurons contain dopamine and it has been shown that this monoamine (1) reduces the responsiveness and receptive field size of horizontal cells, (2) enhances center-responsiveness of the bipolar cells, (3) decreases surround antagonism in bipolar and receptor cells, and (4) depolarizes certain amacrine cells. This suggests that the interplexiform cells modify lateral inhibitory effects mediated by horizontal and amacrine cells and may regulate the strength of center-surround antagonism in retinal neurons. (Interplexiform cells have been recorded intracellularly only rarely; thus their responses are not included in Figure 2.)

Figure 1, in addition to showing the overall cellular organization of the retina, also provides a somewhat speculative summary of the chemical synaptic interactions in the retina and how the major types of ganglion cell receptive fields, i.e.,

on- and off-center and on-off movement-sensitive, may be formed. This scheme reflects mainly cone receptor pathways; less is known concerning rod pathways in the retina. In this diagram, excitatory and inhibitory synapses are indicated by open (excitatory) or closed (inhibitory) circles on the postsynaptic side of the junction. In the retina, however, because many cells respond to light by hyperpolarizing, it is often not easy to decide whether a synapse is excitatory or inhibitory. Thus, a synapse indicated as excitatory means that the postsynaptic response is of the same polarity as the response in the presynaptic element or that the postsynaptic response is enhanced as a result of the synaptic interaction. Conversely, a synapse indicated as inhibitory represents a situation where the postsynaptic response is of opposite polarity to that in the presynaptic element or where the postsynaptic response is diminished as a result of synaptic action. Known reciprocal interactions between two elements, i.e., horizontal cells and cones and certain amacrine cells and bipolar terminals, are also indicated (open triangles).

According to the scheme of Figure 1, cone photoreceptors in the outer plexiform layer make excitatory synapses onto hyperpolarizing bipolar cells and inhibitory synapses onto depolarizing bipolar cells. Reciprocal (forward-excitatory, back inhibitory) synapses occur between cones and horizontal cells, while rods make excitatory synapses onto horizontal cells. Horizontal cells, in turn, make inhibitory synapses onto hyperpolarizing bipolar cells (i.e., they depolarize them) and excitatory synapses onto depolarizing bipolar cells (i.e., they hyperpolarize them). The interplexiform cells make inhibitory synapses onto the horizontal cells, and since they enhance the center responsiveness of both kinds of bipolar cells, the synapses from interplexiform cells to bipolar cells are indicated as excitatory.

In the inner plexiform layer, the bipolar cell terminals make excitatory synapses onto both sustained and transient amacrine cell processes and onto ganglion cell processes. The hyperpolarizing bipolar terminals are found mainly in the upper half of the inner plexiform layer while the depolarizing bipolars are found mainly in the lower half of this layer. Thus a lamination exists in the inner plexiform layer such that off activity is generated principally in the outer part of the layer and on activity in the inner half of the layer. Some synapses between bipolar terminals and amacrine cell processes are reciprocal (shown here between the bipolar cells and transient amacrines). Amacrine cells make mainly inhibitory synapses onto ganglion cells; the well-established exception is the excitatory synapses made by certain transient amacrine cells onto the on-off ganglion cells. In the inner plexiform layer it is supposed that the interplexiform cells receive and make excitatory-like synapses onto transient amacrine cells.

In addition to chemical synapses in the retina, there are also electrical synapses observed in both plexiform layers, which are not represented in Figure 1. These involve mainly the receptor, horizontal, and amacrine cells. Most is known about the electrical junctions between the horizontal cells, which serve to extend the receptive field size of these cells. That is, because of the electrical coupling between the horizontal cells, the receptive field size of the cells is many times larger than the process spread of an individual horizontal cell.

Pharmacology

Knowledge of the synaptic mechanisms and transmitters used in the retina is quite incomplete and under active investigation. Studies of the electrical properties of horizontal and bipolar cells in a variety of retinas suggests that photoreceptors release a depolarizing neurotransmitter in the dark, probably L-glutamate or a similar acidic amino acid, and that light decreases this transmitter flow. High levels of extracellular Mg^{2+} and Co^{2+}, like light, hyperpolarize horizontal cells and hyperpolarizing bipolars, findings consistent with this hypothesis. The evidence thus indicates that many of the distal retinal neurons are active in the dark and that light turns them off. Some horizontal cells in some species appear to use gamma-aminobutyric acid (GABA) as their transmitter, but elsewhere in the outer plexiform layer, information concerning the transmitters used is fragmentary.

In the inner plexiform layer, five classic neurotransmitters (acetylcholine, GABA, glycine, dopamine, and an indoleamine, probably serotonin) and at least seven peptides (somatostatin, substance P, enkephalin, neurotensin, vasoactive intestinal peptide, cholecystokinin, and glucagon) have been associated with amacrine cells. Thus, there are anatomically and pharmacologically distinct subtypes of amacrine cells, which have different synaptic connections and presumably mediate different functions. For example, amacrines releasing acetylcholine appear to provide the excitatory input for on-off movement-sensitive ganglion cells, while amacrine cells releasing GABA provide inhibitory input into on-off, and perhaps on-center ganglion cells. Glycine-releasing amacrine cells also appear to provide major inhibitory input to certain ganglion cells, perhaps mainly off-center cells, while dopamine may play a modulatory role on horizontal, bipolar, and amacrine cells in the retina. Little is known at present about the function of the peptidergic amacrine cells and of possible bipolar cell transmitters.

In summary, the outer plexiform layer of the retina is concerned mainly with the static and spatial aspects of illumination. The neurons contributing processes to that layer respond primarily with sustained, graded potentials, and the neuronal interactions there accentuate contrast in the retinal image by forming an antagonistic center-surround organization at the level of the bipolar cells. The on- and off-center ganglion cells, receiving much of their input directly from either the center-depolarizing or center-hyperpolarizing bipolar cells, reflect this basic center-surround receptive field organization established in the outer plexiform layer. The inner plexiform layer, on the other hand, is concerned more with the dynamic or temporal aspects of photic stimuli. Transient amacrine and the on-off ganglion cells accentuate the changes in retinal illumination and respond vigorously to moving stimuli. Interactions in the inner plexiform layer underlie the motion and directional-selective responses of the on-off ganglion cells.

Further reading

Dowling, JE (1987): *The Vertebrate Retina: An Approachable Part of the Brain*. Cambridge: Harvard Univ. Press

Dowling JE, Dubin MW (1984): The vertebrate retina. In: *Handbook of Physiology, The Nervous System, Vol. III, Sensory Processes,* Darian-Smith I, ed. Baltimore: Williams and Wilkins

Kaneko A (1979): Physiology of the retina. *Ann Rev Neurosci* 2:169–191

Rodieck RW (1973): *The Vertebrate Retina*. San Francisco: WH Freeman

Schmitt FO, Worden FG, eds. (1979): *The Neurosciences: Fourth Study Program*. Cambridge: MIT Press

Retinal Ganglion Cells

Mark Wm. Dubin

Ganglion cells typically make up the innermost layer of the vertebrate retina. They are the only cells with axons that leave the eye. These axons form the optic nerve. Ganglion cell dendrites ramify in the inner nuclear layer, where they are postsynaptic to bipolar cells, which provide a direct input pathway from the outer plexiform layer, and to amacrine cells, which mediate spatially lateral interactions. Via these inputs, each ganglion cell is linked to a roughly circular patch of photoreceptors that subtend a view of space ranging from minutes to degrees of solid angle; the actual size of the field of view depends upon retinal position and animal species. The region in space in which a visual stimulus can substantively influence the firing of a particular ganglion cell is referred to as its receptive field. The network of synaptically linked neurons that define a ganglion cell's receptive field leads to excitatory and inhibitory interactions that are the basis of the cell's being more responsive to certain visual stimuli than to others.

In any one species there are typically a small number of receptive field types, usually named for their visual parameters. For example, one of the most common is the ON-center type. Such fields have a central region that, when illuminated by a spot of light, causes the ganglion cell to respond with a burst of action potentials. Beyond this central region is a concentric surround region that causes a burst of action potentials when light impinging upon it is turned off. The center and surround regions are antagonistic, such that a large stimulus falling on both the center and surround elicits a weaker response both at light onset and offset than would be caused by stimulation of the center or surround alone. Complementary to this receptive field type is the OFF-center ganglion cell in which the responses to center and surround stimulation for the ON-center type are exactly reversed.

ON-center and OFF-center types can be further subdivided in some species by the way in which they summate light falling within their receptive field. In the so-called X-type ganglion cells this summation is spatially linear, such that the effect of adding light in one part of the field can be cancelled by subtracting light in another part. For example, a null position line can be found bisecting the receptive field such that, if light is simultaneously turned off on one side of the field and turned on on the other side, the cell will not substantively respond. In the nonlinear Y-type ganglion cells, no such stimulus change can be made without causing the cell to respond, no matter how carefully a null position is sought. This leads to four different receptive field types, ON-X, OFF-X, ON-Y, OFF-Y, that have been defined most clearly in the cat and in primates. In many species it has been shown that ON-center and OFF-center type ganglion cells have dendrites that ramify in different, nonoverlapping sublayers of the inner plexiform layer, thus receiving inputs from different classes of bipolar and amacrine cells. Similarly, there is a clear and distinct difference between the dendritic morphology of

X-type and Y-type ganglion cells. Such morphological differences are typically a common feature of ganglion cells that have different receptive field types.

In some species, such as goldfish and monkey, ganglion cell receptive fields are color coded. For example, in a concentric type ganglion cell the center may be most sensitive to a red wavelength and the surround to a green wavelength. More complicated, double-opponent color cells exist in which, for example, the center is ON-red, OFF-green, and the surround is OFF-red, ON-green.

In many species, especially among nonmammals, there are numerous nonconcentric type receptive fields. A number of these respond to a spot of light with a burst of impulses at both the onset and cessation of illumination, and hence are known as ON-OFF ganglion cells. A common receptive field of this kind is the direction-selective type. Such a cell responds best to a target moving in a particular direction and not at all to the same target moving in the 180 degree opposite direction (the null direction). This selectivity is independent of stimulus contrast; it is the same for a dark target moving against a light background as for a light target moving on a dark background. Similarly, the directional preference of the cell is not a function of target speed or size. In a species with such direction-selective receptive fields, there is usually a range of cells such that all directions are represented, although certain ones may be most heavily represented. It has been shown that the direction selectivity results from a lateral spread of inhibition in the null direction when a target is moving in that direction, most likely mediated by amacrine cells.

Other types of nonconcentric receptive fields include cells that respond best to targets of a particular size (angular subtense) moving at a particular velocity. In the pigeon, receptive fields in which the best stimulus is a horizontally or vertically oriented moving edge have been reported. In general, such specializations are organized by a network of amacrine connections in the inner plexiform layer. Further, a greater preponderance of nonconcentric receptive field types is present in the retinas of vertebrates such as amphibians, reptiles, and birds than in mammals. In the latter, concentric types predominate. A concentric type receptive field may be thought of as relatively simple compared to the direction-selective type, given that the latter abstracts features from the visual image to a greater degree than does a concentric unit. In the lower vertebrates, with relatively small amounts of brain devoted to vision, it appears that the retina must deal with the visual image more fully—using nonconcentric, specialized type receptive fields—than in higher vertebrates that have an extensive visual cortex where visual processing occurs in a sophisticated fashion.

Initially in the cat, nonconcentric type ganglion cells and certain concentric types were lumped together under the heading W-cell to distinguish them from X-type and Y-type ganglion cells. This terminology has been extended to other species as well. It should be clear that W-cell is strictly a term of convenience, however, and that there is no single W-type receptive field.

In any one species, it is often found that different receptive field types project to different central visual regions. For example, X-type, Y-type, and W-cells in the cat have different patterns of projection to the layers of the lateral geniculate nucleus and to the superior colliculus. Such projection differences are just one of a number of distinguishing features of a receptive field type. It is important to realize that together with morphological and physiological characteristics these features define types that are truly distinct in any particular vertebrate species.

Further reading

Dowling JE, Dubin MW (1984): The vertebrate retina. In: *Handbook of Physiology, The Nervous System, Vol III, Sensory Processes,* Darian-Smith I, ed. Baltimore: Williams and Wilkens

Rodieck RW (1973): *The Vertebrate Retina.* San Francisco: WH Freeman

Stell WK (1972): The morphological organization of the vertebrate retina. In: *Physiology of Photoreceptor Organs,* Fourtes MGF, ed. Berlin: Springer-Verlag

Wässle H (1982): Morphological types and central projections of ganglion cells in the cat retina. In: *Progress in Retinal Research,* Osborne N and Chader G, eds. Oxford: Pergamon Press

Retinotectal Interactions

S.C. Sharma

The ability of fishes and amphibia to regenerate the severed optic nerve has provided investigators with a tool for studying the forces controlling the formation of topographic projections. Initially it had been assumed that regeneration recapitulates development, and the rules governing regeneration would therefore be similar to those governing development. It is clear that formation of orderly connections during development or regeneration depends upon the emergence of specific interactions between optic axons and the tectal neurons. In an effort to explain how regenerating optic axons form specific connections, Roger Sperry postulated that populations of interconnecting neurons each acquire positionally dependent chemoselective labels and that these labels on the optic axons become matched with those of their appropriate target neurons in the tectum. This hypothesis, which has been at times referred to as the chemospecific hopothesis, has served as the basis of extensive experimentation. It has been shown that regenerating optic fibers from a specific part of the retina would grow past an empty area of the optic tectum to terminate in the appropriate portion. Recent evidence supporting the notion of selectivity in the reformation of specific connections indicates the ability of regenerating axons to seek out (1) appropriate recognition of the target areas when confronted with translocated grafts of tectal tissue, resulting in the possibility that affinity markers exist on the tectal cells, and (2) appropriate, albeit normal, connection formation in a rotated and regrafted piece of tectal tissue leading to the formation of a rotated visuotopic map.

In the past 20 years, concerted efforts have been made to deal specifically with the question of whether matching of retinal and tectal markers accounts for the selectivity of the final connections. Size disparity experiments, initially performed by Sperry, gave results in support of such a notion, i.e., regenerating fibers from the half retina terminate only on the appropriate tectal zone immediately after regeneration. However, six months following initial surgery, the half retinal projection begins to expand while maintaining retinotopic order and finally covers the whole *tectum*. The size disparity experiments involving the partial ablation of the tectum following optic nerve crush have led to similar results (i.e., initial normal map from the appropriate half retinal area and subsequent compression of the complete visuotopic field onto the remaining half tectum). The expansion of the half retinal map and the compression of the complete map onto the half tectum have been incorporated under the term neuronal plasticity. The idea that retinal axons would form connections only with the appropriate target center was refuted by the above experiments, which suggest that retinotectal connections are labile. However, regardless of the particular stage of regeneration, retinotopic order is maintained.

In order to explain lability in retinotopic connections during regeneration, various hypotheses have been proposed: (1) Reti-notopic order emerges from the positional markers on the retinal fibers whereby axons in the nerve develop topographic order by maintaining neighborhood relationships in the optic pathway. (2) The orientation of the map on the tectum requires both polarity information on the brain tissue and imprinting of axonal label onto the tectal cells. (3) Competition exists among regenerating axons for formation of specific synapses while maintaining retinotopic order. (4) Affinity markers are present on the tectum, as shown by the stability of the map following tectal tissue translocations.

Each of these hypotheses has been under extensive experimentation, and each may explain only certain aspects of known specificity. Perhaps all such hypotheses together may explain both specificity and lability of connections in the retinotectal system. The major drawback in most proposed hypotheses seems to be that they are not easily testable.

Morphologically, information relevant to understanding the compression phenomenon has recently emerged. During regeneration, the optic nerve transiently innervates the wrong pathways, suggesting a trial-and-error process in successful reinnervation of the proper target. Large numbers of exploratory axons do not associate with degenerating debris or glia, and the first phase of regeneration is that of diffuse exploratory growth. In the presence of the target tissue, the number of exploratory branches increases 5–10-fold. Hence, the role of target tissue appears to be in the maintenance of early fascicles and the promotion of subsequent growth. This diffuse projection of axons may suggest the earlier phase of regeneration during which the retinotopic map is rather poor. The maturation of the appropriate projection is followed by the retraction of inappropriate axonal branches. During the compression following half tectal ablation, the regenerating axons compete for limited accommodation on the target neurons. The postsynaptic cells only accept the normal number of synapses. Thus, in compression each regenerating axon eventually has a decreased number of synaptic terminals. If one assumes that one optic axon has two branches and two synapses in normal condition, during compression each axon will now only have half the normal number. With this mechanism, the postsynaptic densities of each tectal cell will remain constant.

In these situations, the number of ganglion cells in the retina does not decrease, nor is there any increase in the dendritic arbor of tectal neurons. The temporal sequence of these changes during compression compares favorably with both electrophysiological and behavioral studies.

Following compression of the visual field onto the half tectum, subsequent changes occur in tectal efferent centers. One good example is the change in the isthmotectal and tectoisthmal projections. The normal topographically ordered projection between the nucleus isthmi and the tectum changes following half tectal ablation and visuotopic compression. The resultant topographic projection between the isthmus and the tectum is ordered. There is expansion of the tectal projection to the isthmus and a comparable compression of the isthmic projection to the tectum. These compensatory changes may be a prerequisite for the return of normal behavior. The factors that control the tectoisthmic projections are not yet well understood.

Efforts are currently under way to discover the molecular basis of retinotectal specificity by immunological and molecular biological techniques. A molecule, which is distributed in a dorsoventral gradient, has been extracted from the chick retina, but it is not clear whether this molecule has any specific role in terms of cellular markers on the ganglion cell. Another molecule is N-CAM for which a role in retinotectal specificity has been implicated. Precisely how these molecules are involved in determining retinotectal specificity may become evident in future studies.

In conclusion, it is safe to assume that retinotectal specificity is not based on a specific molecule that exhibits a lock-and-key mechanism. Such a conclusion is supported by the size disparity experiments. Future research should be directed toward understanding how a single identifiable axon forms connections in this system and the molecular basis of recognition between the retina and the tectum. This may perhaps elucidate the understanding of the formation of patterned neural connections.

Further reading

Edwards MA, Sharma SC, Murray M (1985): Selective retinal innervation of a surgically created tectal island in goldfish. I. Light microscopic analysis. *J Comp Neurol* 232:372–385

Dunn-Meynell AA, Sharma SC (1984): Changes in the topographically organized connections between the nucleus isthmi and the optic tectum after partial tectal ablation in adult goldfish. *J Comp Neurol* 227:497–510

Murray M, Sharma SC, Edwards MA (1982): Target regulation of synaptic number in the compressed retinotectal projection of goldfish. *J Comp Neurol* 209:374–385

Schmidt JT (1982): The formation of retinotectal projections. *Trends Neurosci* 5:111–116

Sharma SC, Romeskie M (1984): Plasticity of retinotectal connections in teleosts. In: *Comparative Neurology of the Optic Tectum*, Vanegas H, ed. New York: Plenum Press

Stereopsis, Binocular Perception

John P. Frisby

Due to their different positions, the two eyes in general receive slightly different images of the world. Differences between left and right images are termed binocular disparities and the human visual system, as well as those of many other species, can detect and use these disparities to recover information about the three-dimensional structure of the scene being viewed. Stereopsis is the term used to describe the perception of depth from binocular disparities.

A stimulus point can be so positioned that it has zero binocular disparity, i.e., it projects to exactly corresponding retinal coordinates in the two eyes. The locus of all such points is termed the point horopter. For a fixation point nearer than infinity, this horopter is a single tilted line passing through the fixation point, together with a circle lying in a horizontal plane passing through the fixation point and the optical centers of the two eyes. Any point not lying on the point horopter projects with either a vertical disparity, or with both a vertical and a horizontal disparity, between its left and right eye image coordinates. Vertical disparities are mainly produced by points (lying off the horizontal plane) that are nearer one eye than the other (as when a point is viewed with an off-center angle of gaze) and whose vertical distance from the horizontal meridian thus projects with a different size in the two eyes. Horizontal disparities arise when a point lies in front or behind the plane of the fixation point, in which case they are termed crossed (or convergent) and uncrossed (or divergent) disparities, respectively, although horizontal disparities are also produced by off-center gaze. Both horizontal and vertical disparities have a component due to eccentricity of retinal location, and both are usually expressed quantitatively as the angle subtended by the difference in coordinates between the left and right images.

The disparity resolution of the human visual system is remarkably fine, optimal conditions producing 75% discrimination of a horizontal disparity of about 2 arc sec so that for a viewing distance of 25 cm, perceptions of depth differences of about 25 μm are possible. It is commonly stated that for viewing distances greater than a few meters, binocular disparities are too small to be detectable, but this is false, as can readily be appreciated by comparing monocular and binocular viewing of landscapes containing large depth differences between objects sited a long distance away.

Points with small horizontal binocular disparities produce the percept of a single entity (providing also that their vertical disparities are small) lying in a depth plane different from that of the fixation point. Such points are thus said to produce binocular fusion and stereoscopic depth, with the size of the perceived depth difference being proportional to the size of the disparity. The range of disparities over which a stimulus in one eye can be presented in order to provide fusion with the same stimulus in the other eye is termed Panum's fusional area. This area is elliptical in shape, with the vertical disparity

limit being smaller than the horizontal, but its dimensions are determined by many factors, e.g., stimulus texture and size (large stimuli with rich textures give largest values); retinal eccentricity (larger values in periphery); and recent history of stimulation (once fused, a richly textured stimulus can remain fused for disparities larger than Panum's limit for initial fusion. If disparity is increased beyond Panum's area the first loss is fusion, with doubled or diplopic images being seen in depth. Further increase in disparity produces diplopia without depth. Disparate points lying outside Panum's area are dealt with by the visual system generating a suitable change in eye positions to reduce the disparity and bring the points within range of Panum's area for the new fixation. An important recent refinement, due to Burt, Julesz, and Tyler, of the notion of Panum's fusional area concerns disparity gradient: if two fused points with different disparities are brought closer and closer together while the disparity between them is maintained, there comes a point when if the disparity gradient between them exceeds a certain limit (about 1.0 for human vision) then one or other of the points is seen diplopic however small the absolute disparity difference between points.

Theoretical problems in understanding stereopsis can be divided into two main categories: disparity measurement and disparity interpretation. The critical problem in disparity measurement is selecting the correct matches between points (sometimes called matching primitives) extracted from the two images. Usually many possibilities are theoretically possible, most of them false. Study of this problem has been considerably advanced using random-dot stereograms in which the disparity signal exists only as a correlation between random texture noise fields sent to each eye, thereby excluding all other cues to depth. Progress in understanding ways of solving the correspondence problem has now reached a stage where successful computer implementations of principled solutions are within reach.

Random-dot stereograms demonstrate that the correspondence problem can be solved at a very early stage of visual processing (i.e., no reliance on complex object recognition processes is necessary). Hence, it is not surprising that neurophysiological studies of binocular vision have demonstrated that neurons responding appropriately to dynamic random-dot stereograms can be found at the earliest stages of binocular interaction in cortical area 17 in the macaque. Exactly how those neurons are computing a solution to the correspondence problem is, however, as yet unclear. The answer will require neurophysiological studies cast within the framework of the computational approach to vision e.g., as advanced by Marr.

The major problem in the interpretation of measured disparities has always been regarded as their intrinsically ambiguous nature (e.g., a given disparity might be produced by a large depth difference viewed from a great distance, or by a small depth difference seen from near at hand). Clarifying this ambiguity has been assumed to require other information about viewing distance in order to scale the disparity measurements (e.g., the extraretinal information about eye vergence angle, cf, some optical rangefinders). It is now known, however, that vertical disparities, hitherto usually regarded simply as an impediment to the efficient use of horizontal disparities, can yield the crucial information about viewing distance (and angle of gaze) that enables the otherwise ambiguous horizontal disparities to be scaled appropriately to recover both the relative and absolute depths of all points within the scene.

About 2–4% of the population do not possess stereopsis, often being unaware of their deficiency until it is revealed by routine clinical stereopsis screening tests, available from distributors of optometric equipment. The development of binocular vision and its susceptibility to disruption by squints and other phenomena has a large psychophysical and neurophysiological literature.

Further reading

Julesz RJ (1971): *Foundations of Cyclopean Perception.* Chicago: University of Chicago Press

Marr D (1982): *Vision.* San Francisco: WH Freeman

Poggio GF, Poggio T (1984): The analysis of stereopsis. *Ann Rev Neurosci* 7:379–412

Pollard SB, Mayhew JEW, Frisby JP (1985): PMF: A stereo correspondence algorithm using a disparity gradient limit. *Perception* 14:449–470

Tyler CW, Scott AR (1981): Binocular vision. In: *Physiology of the Human Eye and Visual System,* Record RE, ed. London: Harper & Row

Strabismus: Ocular Malalignment

Theodore Lawwill

Strabismus is a clinical condition of the eyes where the visual axes of the two eyes are not both directed at the object of regard. The common deviation is "crossed eyes" (esotropia). While most strabismus has its onset in infancy or the first two years of life, adult onset does occur in association with neurological and vascular disease or trauma. Under normal circumstances the two eyes are under exquisite control with the visual axes aligned within a few seconds of arc by the six extraocular muscles of each eye. Several neurological inputs including the vestibular system and neck proprioceptive signals serve to align the eyes even without visual feedback. The final alignment is locked in when the two eyes are operating together, fusing into a single image the signals from corresponding points from the two eyes.

Strabismus may occur on a mechanical, neurological, or anatomical basis. Often there is a combination of factors as in the case of accommodative esotropia. Individuals with accommodative esotropia are farsighted (hyperopic). Being farsighted means that they must use their accommodative (near focusing) power even to focus in the distance. For every amount of accommodation made a corresponding convergence (turning in) effort is produced. The only reason a nonstrabismic hyperope has straight eyes is that he has strong fusion, and the strong cortical visual feedback overcomes the excessive convergence effort. The accommodative esotrope just does not have the fusional reserve. Interestingly this lack of fusional reserve can often be demonstrated in family members who do not have hyperopia or esotropia. A majority of accommodative esotropes can be corrected by wearing glasses that correct the hyperopia. In some cases of strabismus, particularly when the eyes turn out (exotropia), the deviation can be intermittent with the eyes sometimes deviated and sometimes straight. Vertical deviations (hypertropias) occur both alone and in association with horizontal deviations. Cyclorotary deviations on the anterior-posterior axis (cyclotropias) occur less frequently but can be quite troublesome.

The six muscles to the eye include four rectus muscles that turn the eye in, out, up, and down. These muscles also have lesser amounts of cyclorotary effect, depending upon the position of the eye. The elevators and depressors also have a small adducting (in) effect. Two cyclorotary muscles basically intort and extort the eye, but they also have significant depressor and elevator effects. The third, fourth, and sixth cranial nerves innervate the extraocular muscles. The sixth, the abducens, supplies the lateral rectus, which abducts (turns out) the eye. The fourth supplies the superior oblique muscle, which incyclorotates the eye. The rest are supplied by the superior and inferior branches of the third oculomotor nerve. The nuclei for these cranial nerves are located along the two sides of the midline in the midbrain. They are interconnected by the median longitudinal fasciculus and receive input from the lateral gaze center located more laterally in the pons. Vestibular, spinal, cerebellar, and cortical input are all important for the movement and final position of the eyes. Imbalances in this system cause malalignment of the visual axes, or strabismus.

Tropia and phoria

When the eyes are given an opportunity to work together and there is a manifest deviation of the axes, a tropia is said to be present. When this deviation is intermittent, an intermittent tropia is present. When fusion is not allowed, as when one eye is covered, the deviation the eyes assume is called a phoria. The phoria may be large or small and is not necessarily pathological. Some phoria is normal as can be demonstrated by looking at a distant object and slowly covering first one eye and then the other, not letting the two work together. The apparent movement of the object is proportional to the deviation under cover or the phoria. Phorias that are large in proportion to fusional reserve can cause eye strain.

Adult-onset strabismus occurs in such diseases as diabetes where the small vessels to the nerves that innervate the extraocular muscles are occluded. Thyroid ophthalmopathy causes infiltration and swelling of the extraocular muscles and restriction of ocular rotation, thus causing strabismus. Injuries can interrupt the innervation or can interfere directly with the function of the muscles.

When strabismus begins in childhood, double vision might be experienced for a while, but soon the offending image is suppressed either in one eye all the time or in either eye alternately. Constant unilateral suppression at a young age leads to strabismic amblyopia, the loss of visual acuity in one eye due to suppression. Adult-onset strabismus often leads to intractable diplopia.

In instances where the alignment is not too far off, sometimes correction can be achieved by wearing prisms in glasses to correct the deviation. In other cases surgical correction may be attempted. Unfortunately, the only surgical procedures available move the muscles on the globe to shorten or lengthen them, and thus do not directly attack the problem, which is more often the imbalance in the innervation to the muscles.

Present understanding of strabismus in its many forms, origins, and ages of onset is based on clinical experience. The complexity of the oculomotor system is sufficient to impede complete understanding even of the kinetic system of saccades and pursuit movements. Conjugate static position and vergences are understood only superficially. Therapy is limited to exercise to strengthen whatever sensory system integration is available and gross alteration of the muscles by surgically moving them or injecting *Botulinum* toxin into them. A greater understanding of the integration of the sensory and motor systems and individual variations may lead to more precise methods of treatment of strabismus in the future.

Further reading

Von Noorden GK, Burian HM (1979): *Burian-von Noorden's Binocular Vision and Ocular Motility: Theory and Management of Strabismus*, 2nd ed. St. Louis: CV Mosby

Striate Cortex

Peter H. Schiller

The striate cortex is an expanse of cortical tissue that in higher mammals comprises a large portion of the occipital lobe. Transverse sections of this tissue, when stained (e.g., with cresyl violet), reveal a distinct striation in layer 4 of its multiple laminae, called the stripe of Gennary; this stripe is not evident in other cortical areas. Six major laminae have been identified, spanning a thickness of approximately 2 mm of gray matter, which have been further divided into several sublaminae. In primates the striate cortex is the major recipient zone of the input from the dorsal lateral geniculate nucleus of the thalamus; fibers terminate most profusely in layer 4c which has two subdivisions, 4c alpha and 4c beta. In primates the projections to 4c alpha and beta originate from the magnocellular and parvocellular divisions of the lateral geniculate nucleus, respectively, and represent two distinct information processing channels originating in the retina, which in Old World monkeys have been identified as the color-opponent and broad-band channels. There are also less dense projections from the lateral geniculate nucleus to layers 1 and 6. The striate cortex makes extensive connections with several extrastriate regions; these projections originate predominantly in layers dorsal to 4c. Projections to subcortical areas, including the thalamus and the midbrain, originate predominantly in layers 5 and 6.

The visual field is represented in an orderly manner on the surface of the striate cortex, with more tissue allocated for central than for the peripheral vision. Each cell is sensitive to only a small region of the visual field, the receptive field area of the cell. Further specificity exists for the stimuli that appear within the receptive field as cells respond selectively to various stimulus dimensions. This specificity becomes greatly elaborated in the striate cortex as compared with the lateral geniculate nucleus. Six major new attributes appear in the population of single cells residing in the striate cortex: (1) Selectivity for the orientation of line segments, (2) selectivity for the direction of stimulus movement, (3) selectivity for the spatial frequency of repetitive stimuli such as textures, (4) double color-opponent color selectivity, (5) sensitivity for both light increment (on response) and light decrement (off response), and (6) binocular activation which for some cells originates from disparate retinal areas, thereby providing information for stereoscopic depth perception. In the primate these attributes are not evident in layers 4c alpha and beta where most cells are similar to those found in the lateral geniculate nucleus.

In addition to its laminar arrangement, the striate cortex is also organized in a columnar fashion. This organization is complex and not yet clearly understood. It has been demonstrated that the orientation specificity and the ocular dominance distributions of single cells form distinct columns in several but not all species. Columnar organization has also been demonstrated for spatial frequency and color selectivity. Figure 1 shows one current model for the organization of the striate cortex of the rhesus monkey. According to this model orientation and ocular dominance columns are arranged orthogonally with respect to each other; cell groups without orientation specificity form rod-like regions inserted at regular intervals in the columns. Among the group of orientation-specific cells, several different classes have been discerned, which include the so-called simple and complex cells. The receptive fields

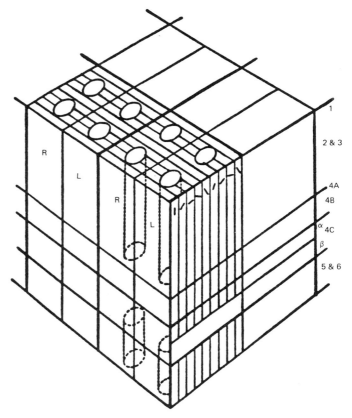

Figure 1. A current model of the striate cortex as proposed by M. S. Livingstone and D. H. Hubel. Columns are shown for ocular dominance (L = left eye; R = right eye) and for orientation (columnar specificity is indicated by the orientation of the line segments drawn at the edge of each column). The rod-like regions represent areas dominated by unoriented cells, many of which are color selective. These regions in histological sections can be selectively labeled with cytochrome oxidase. Cortical layers are numbered on the right. Four modules as shown, two in detail. From Livingston MS, Hubel DH (1984): Anatomy and physiology of a color system in the primate visual cortex. *J. Neuroscience* 4:309–356.

of simple cells subdivide into spatially separate regions, within each of which responses are selective for either light increment (on response) or light decrement (off response). Complex cells, which commonly receive input from both eyes, do not exhibit such subdivisions; they typically respond to both light increment and decrement throughout their receptive fields.

The experimental evidence gathered indicates that the striate cortex is modular. Each module performs the same analysis but deals with a different portion of visual space. A module is approximately $1 \times 1 \times 2$ mm and contains a full cycle of orientations and ocular dominances as shown in Figure 1. Based on inputs from thalamic centers as well as feedback information from other cortical areas, each module is capable of analyzing the pattern, wavelength, luminance, movement, and depth of visual stimuli appearing in the visual field. This information is then relayed for further analysis to other cortical centers as well as to subcortical ones.

The basic organization of the striate cortex appears to be genetically determined. However, the impact of the environment can dramatically alter its makeup. It has been shown that when animals are deprived of vision through one eye during early life, dramatic reorganization occurs. After such deprivation the neurons of the striate cortex can no longer be activated by the deprived eye. Columns representing the deprived eye shrink and columns representing the normal eye expand. Behavioral studies show pronounced deficits in depth perception and pattern perception through the deprived eye. Deficits in neuronal function and in behavior have also been shown in animals which have become strabismic and amblyopic in early life or have been reared in environments lacking information about stimulus motion.

Further reading

Poggio GF (1980): Central neural mechanisms in vision. In: *Medical Physiology*, 14th ed, Mountcastle, VB, ed. St. Louis: CV Mosby

Texture Perception

Bela Julesz

Texture is the fundamental property of visible surfaces. Since objects are covered by surfaces, in order to be visible the surfaces must be textured so that their reflectances cast on our retinae have luminance or color variations. These surface patterns enable us to discriminate between apples and oranges, or find a needle in a haystack. While at some scale all textured surfaces have a three-dimensional relief that can be both visually and tactilely sensed, here we are concerned only with the two-dimensional surface patterns cast on the retinae.

This restriction to two-dimensional patterns does not mean that the textures cannot be perceived in three dimensions. It is still an enigma how the granularity of real-life textures (e.g., the aerial photograph of a plowed field, or a field of grass) can be perceived in depth when viewed by one eye. We know much more how the slant of textured surfaces is perceived based on the retinal gradient of the texture elements as first discussed by J.J. Gibson in 1950. In the case of homogeneous textures, texture gradients are one of the many perspective cues that yield monocular depth information, and abrupt changes in texture gradients give rise to edges and corners.

Understanding texture discrimination has important applications, which range from the breaking of camouflage to automatic texture analysis of the biomedical imagery encountered in pathology, hematology, immunology, genetics, radiology, and nuclear medicine. These applications are based on ad hoc specialized techniques, each having a vast literature. Subsequent to the compilation edited by Lipkin and Rosenfeld in 1970, much of the recent literature on texture analysis for biomedical applications has been reviewed by Pressman and co-workers.

In order to understand human texture discrimination, one must study simplified textures and low-level perceptual modes. This can be done by reducing textures to arrays of synthetic texture elements composed of dots and line segments and by restricting the perceptual mode to preattentive (effortless) texture discrimination in place of the element-by-element scrutiny of attentive discrimination. Julesz and his collaborators have carried out an extensive program of research using these methods. With synthetic textures having controlled statistical properties (e.g., texture pairs with identical first-, second-, third-order statistics), they were able to show that the preattentive human visual system cannot use global (statistical) texture parameters, but instead uses local conspicuous features called textons. Figure 1 shows typical textures composed of line-segment textons of the same length, width, and color (black), thrown at random orientations, but such that two adjacent line segments are perpendicular to each other forming T-, L-, and +-shaped texture elements. The aggregates of +'s effortlessly segregate from the surrounding aggregates of Ls; this preattentive texture segregation is a parallel process, since a single + stands out from the L-shaped surround as fast as many +'s, regardless of their number. On the other hand, it requires element-by-element scrutiny to detect the aggregate of T-shaped elements, even though this aggregate is as large as the one composed of +s. Here one needs a serial process of focal attention (scrutiny).

Textons are elongated blobs (rectangles, ellipses, and line segments) of specific colors, orientations, widths, lengths (and also of binocular disparity, velocity, and flicker rate). In the case of line segments, their crossings and terminations (ends-of-lines) behave as textons, too. The preattentive parallel visual system can detect only texton-gradients where adjacent texture elements differ in their texton number or density. However, the preattentive visual system cannot recognize the positional relationships between textons (i.e., the glue between adjacent textons is missing). Only in a small aperture of focal attention, which can be moved in 20–50-msec steps at will (and is 4–8 times faster than scanning eye movements) can one recognize the spatial relationships among local features that enable the attentive system to perform the prodigious feats of form recognition. Thus, in Figure 1 preattentive texture discrimination is based on the texton of crossing, which is contained in the +'s but is lacking in the Ls. By contrast, the T- and L-shaped elements of Figure 1 are composed of the same textons, and their aggregates cannot be preattentively discriminated. Only in the small aperture of focal attention as we scrutinize the textures element-by-element are we able to tell a T from an L.

Figure 2 gives another illustration of the power of the texton theory. Figure 2A shows a pair of line drawings portraying an S- and 10-shaped element. While in isolation (and while being scrutinized), they appear quite different from each other, one being connected and open, the other having two unconnected parts of which one is closed. It is also apparent that both elements are composed of the same textons (three identical horizontal line segments, two identical vertical line segments, and two line ends). Therefore, according to the texton theory, if scrutiny is prevented, these elements could not yield preattentive texture discrimination. Indeed, a texture pair composed of these two elements (Fig. 2B) cannot be distinguished preattentively. Even a single element embedded in an aggregate of elements composed of the same number of textons cannot be detected without scrutiny. If Figure 2C is presented briefly and the long-persistent afterimage is erased after 100 msec by a masker the S in 10-shaped elements cannot be detected. (However, any change of texton equilibrium would yield preattentive discrimination. For instance, if one of the vertical line segments in the S or 10-shapes in Figure 2A is changed to form an E shape, then the terminator number increases from 2 to 3 and the E can be effortlessly detected among the background of S- or 10-shaped elements.)

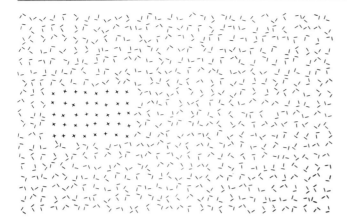

Figure 1. Preattentive texture discrimination is shown between areas composed of +'s and Ls, while element-by-element scrutiny, called focal attention, is required to find the Ts embedded in the Ls. From Julesz and Bergen (1983).

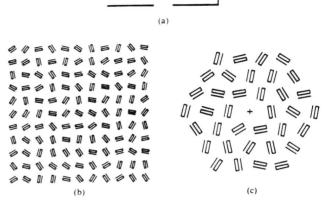

Figure 2. Demonstration of how the heuristics given in text predict why (a) the differently appearing S- and 10-shaped elements in aggregates (b) and one S among 10's (c) are indistinguishable. From Julesz (1981).

The essence of the texton theory is that texton gradients and their locations are immediately detected by the preattentive system, and this knowledge where gradients occur in turn enables the attentive system to examine them one by one and to determine what is located there. Somewhat similar theories have been postulated by Treisman and her co-workers and Marr and his followers in the frameworks of cognitive psychology and artificial intelligence, respectively. The Julesz theory differs from the cognitive theories by emphasizing the short range over which texton gradients can be computed; for elements that are not adequately close to each other, so that no textures are perceived, the texton theory cannot be applied. The Julesz theory also differs from Marr's theory in that the former states that perceptual elements, such as the textons, exist only in preattentive vision, while attentive vision, which can glue the textons together in countless ways to form *Gestalten,* may possess no primitive elements. The texton concept of local conspicuous feature differences among texton pairs having identical statistics up to a high order is very different from the superficially similar feature theories postulated by some other psychologists, even though important contributions were made by them, particularly in textural groupings.

There is a close relation between the notion of textons as revealed by statistically controlled texture pairs using methods of experimental psychology and the local trigger features of Kuffler and of Hubel and Wiesel who found in the visual cortex of cat and monkey neurons that selectively fired for elongated blobs and edges of certain colors, orientations, width, velocity, etc. These feature analyzers appear to be segregated in various visual cortical areas, forming modules (texton pools), as found by Zeki and others. These modules can easily process texton gradients; however, as one moves the searchlight of focal attention to those texton gradients, how the many textons that are extracted in these modules are glued together in exact positional alignment to form shapes is a crucial problem of brain research.

Further reading

Beck JJ (1967): Perceptual grouping produced by line figures. *Percept Psychophys* 2:491–495

Bergen JR, Julesz B (1983): Parallel versus serial processing in rapid pattern discrimination. *Nature* 303:696–698

Caelli T, Julesz B, Gilbert EN (1978): On perceptual analyzers underlying texture discrimination: Part II. *Biol Cybernet* 29(4):201–214

Gibson JJ (1950): *The Perception of the Visual World.* Boston: Houghton Mifflin

Hubel DH, Wiesel TN (1968): Receptive fields and functional architecture of monkey striate cortex. *J Physiol* 195:215–243

Julesz B (1962): Visual pattern discrimination. IRE *Trans Info Theor* IT-8:84–92.

Julesz B (1975): Experiments in the visual perception of texture. *Sci Am* 232(4):34–43

Julesz B (1981): Textons, the elements of texture perception, and their interactions. *Nature* 290:91–97

Julesz B (1984): A brief outline of the texton theory of human vision. *Trends Neurosci* 7:41–45

Julesz B, Gilbert EN, Shepp LA, Frisch HL (1973): Inability of humans to discriminate between visual textures that agree in second-order statistics—revisited. *Perception* 2:391–405

Julesz B, Gilbert EN, Victor JD (1978): Visual discrimination of textures with identical third-order statistics. *Biol Cybernet* 31:137–140

Julesz B, Bergen JR (1983): Textons: The Fundamental Elements in Preattentive Vision and Perception of Textures. *Bell Syst Tech J* 62 (6):1619–1645

Kuffler SW (1953): Discharge patterns and functional organization of mammalian retina. *J Neurophysiol* 16:37–68

Lipkin BS, Rosenfeld A, eds (1970): *Picture Processing and Psychopictorics.* New York: Academic

Marr D (1982): *Vision.* San Francisco: WH Freeman

Pressman NJ, Haralick RM, Tyrer HW, Frost JK (1979): Texture analysis for biomedical imagery. In: *Biomedical Pattern Recognition and Image Processing,* Fu KS, Pavlidis T, eds. Berlin: Dahlem Konferenzen

Treisman A, Gelade G (1980): A feature-integration theory of attention. *Cog Psychol* 12:97–136

Zeki SM (1978): Functional specialisation in the visual cortex of the rhesus monkey. *Nature* 274:423–28

Vision, Deprivation Studies

Nigel W. Daw

Visual deprivation occurs when the optical input to the visual system is restricted in young animals. The visual system, which is still malleable in young animals, responds with alterations in its connections. Thus visual deprivation can lead to permanent alterations in the visual system, which may be deleterious if the normal input is restored.

The best known example of visual deprivation is monocular deprivation. This occurs when one eye is closed or lost, or when the image on the retina of one eye is so degraded that no contours are seen. The behavioral effects of monocular deprivation were noticed late in the 19th century when surgical removal of the lens for cataract became common. In patients with unilateral cataract, where the whole of the lens of one eye was cloudy, so that no images could be seen in that eye, the results of the surgery depended on the age of the patient. Adults who developed cataracts were improved by the surgery—their sight was restored. People who had a congenital cataract removed were not helped—they could not see well (a condition called amblyopia) through the eye that had had the surgery, even if they used artificial lenses to produce a perfectly good image on the retina. These results demonstrated two points: first, that some part of the nervous system behind the photoreceptors may be altered; and second, that there is a critical period early in life during which the alterations occur.

The anatomical and physiological basis for these observations was worked out in a series of experiments started by David Hubel and Torsten Wiesel in the early 1960s. Hubel and Wiesel worked with young cats and macaque monkeys and sutured the lids of one eye shut to produce monocular deprivation. They then opened the eye and recorded from a sample of cells in the visual cortex and found that nearly all the cells were dominated by the eye that had remained open; very few cells could be driven through the eye that had been closed. The strength of the effect depended on the age of the animal and the duration of the eyelid suture. At the peak of the critical period, which is 4–5 weeks of age for kittens, the effect could be surprisingly strong: one or two days of eyelid suture could produce large shifts in eye dominance for the cells in the visual cortex.

The part of the system that is mainly affected by monocular deprivation is the primary visual cortex. The input to the visual cortex comes from the lateral geniculate body, with endings in layer IV of the cortex (Fig. 1). In normal cats and monkeys these endings lie in alternating strips, one set of strips for the left eye and one set of strips for the right eye. Most cells in layers above and below the endings receive input from both sets of strips, so that they are binocularly driven. After the left eye has been sutured closed for a suitable period, the area covered by the endings from the left eye is smaller than normal, and the area covered by endings from the right eye is larger than normal. This is part of the reason why most cells in the visual cortex are dominated by the open eye.

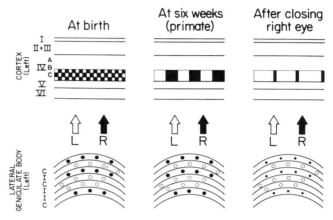

Figure 1. Normal development and effects of monocular deprivation in the visual system of the macaque. In the normal macaque the geniculocortical endings in layer IV C of the cortex segregate between birth and six weeks of age, until alternate strips are seen. (There are also endings in layers IV A and VI, but the effect is most noticeable in layer IV C.) After closing the right eye at birth, cells in geniculate layers receiving input from that eye (layers 1, 4, and 6, counting from the bottom) become smaller. The endings of those cells in layer IV C of the cortex are substantially reduced. Geniculate layers marked C are innervated by the contralateral (right) eye: those marked I are innervated by the ipsilateral (left) eye.

Other parts of the visual system are also affected. Primary visual cortex projects on to secondary visual cortex and subcortical areas such as the superior colliculus. Cells in those areas are also dominated by the open eye. The physiological properties of cells in the lateral geniculate nucleus are not affected much. However, these cells provide support for their endings in the cortex, and the cells with fewer endings are smaller (Fig. 1).

Some of the changes in the visual cortex resulting from monocular deprivation occur because the normal process of development of the visual cortex is disrupted. This can be seen most clearly in the macaque monkey. At birth, the endings from the two eyes in layer IV of the visual cortex are mingled together. Over the first six weeks of life these endings reform and segregate from each other until the adult pattern of alternating strips is seen. This probably occurs through a process of competition between inputs from the two eyes for synaptic space on the postsynaptic neuron. If one eye (the right, for example) is sutured shut at birth, then endings from the right eye retract, while endings from the left eye do not.

There are a variety of different kinds of visual deprivation, each of which leads to a result specific to the deprivation imposed. Animals may be reared in an environment continually moving in one direction (to the right, for example). After this treatment, there is an increased percentage of cells in the visual cortex preferring movement to the right, and a reduced percentage preferring leftward movement.

Animals may also be reared in an environment of stripes all oriented in one direction (vertical, for example). After this treatment there is an increased percentage of cells in the visual cortex preferring vertical orientation, and a reduced percentage preferring horizontal orientation. A related situation occurs in humans with astigmatism, i.e., a cylindrical component to the lens such that contours of one orientation are in focus on the retina while contours of the perpendicular orientation are out of focus. People who have astigmatism as a child have permanently reduced acuity (this is known as meridional amblyopia) for the contours that were out of focus on their retina, even after the astigmatism is corrected by lenses.

In strabismus the two eyes look in different directions because of problems in motor control of the eyes. Strabismus may be esotropic, with one eye turned inward, or exotropic, with one eye turned outward. All strabismics lose binocular vision and functions that depend on binocular vision, such as stereoscopic depth perception. Esotropes compensate for their diplopia (double vision) by losing acuity in one eye. Exotropes generally compensate for their diplopia by using one eye and then the other. The underlying mechanisms for these phenomena can be seen in animals made strabismic by cutting or shortening some eye muscles. In both esotropes and exotropes, very few cells in the visual cortex can be driven by both eyes. In the case of esotropic animals, the acuity of cells in the lateral geniculate body driven by the eye looking inward is probably reduced.

Finally, both eyes may be closed (binocular deprivation). This occurs in children who have bilateral cataract at an early age. The result is poor vision in both eyes. Many cells in the visual cortex are still driven by both eyes, but their responses are poor and many of them cannot be driven by either eye.

Some anatomical and physiological mechanisms underlying monocular deprivation have been discussed. Other mechanisms must be involved in other kinds of visual deprivation, although the specific experiments required to show them have not yet been done. Orientation and direction sensitivity within the visual cortex depend on inhibitory interactions arising from neurons containing gamma-aminobutyric acid (GABA). Changes in orientation and direction sensitivity presumably result from changes in the connections of these GABA neurons. The effects of binocular deprivation, which involve a loss of orientation and direction sensitivity, probably also involve changes in the network of GABA neurons.

The critical period for the effects of visual deprivation varies with the species studied, the kind of visual deprivation used, and the level of the visual system studied. The three species that have been most studied are cats, macaques, and humans. In cats the critical period lasts from around eye opening to three months of age or later. In macaques it involves the first six months of life. In humans it involves the first six years of life. In general the system is most susceptible early in the critical period (four to five weeks for cats, six months to two years for humans) with a steady decline in susceptibility after that. It is important to realize, however, particularly in treating

humans, that a deficit can be alleviated after the critical period for the creation of that deficit is over. For example, closing one eye in a kitten after the age of three months has little effect. However, if an eye is closed before the age of three months, so that the animal is amblyopic in that eye at the age of three months, opening the eye up and possibly closing the other eye at three months can reduce the amblyopia.

The critical period for directional deprivation ends earlier than the critical period for monocular deprivation. Presumably this is because different nerve connections are concerned: binocularity involves convergence of excitatory influences from the two eyes while directional sensitivity involves lateral GABA inhibitory connections within the visual cortex. However, the critical period for the effects of monocular deprivation is not a single period. Three effects of monocular deprivation are: a reduction in the size of some lateral geniculate cells, a reduction in the area in layer IV occupied by endings from the deprived eye, and a change in eye dominance for cells in the visual cortex. The critical period for lateral geniculate cell size ends earlier than the period for endings in layer IV, which ends earlier than the period for dominance in the visual cortex. There are, in fact, two sets of endings in layer IV, and evidence indicates that there are different critical periods for them.

There has been a substantial body of research recently looking for factors that may modulate, alter, or prevent the effects of visual deprivation, or extend the critical period. Hypotheses have been advanced that one of the nonvisual inputs to the visual cortex (mediated by agents such as noradrenaline, acetylcholine, serotonin, or dopamine) may change the effects of visual deprivation, but the evidence is presently controversial. Input from proprioceptors in the eye movement system may play a role. Whether the animal is anesthetized during the period of monocular deprivation certainly does. Activity in the retinogeniculocortical pathway is important, particularly when inputs to the cortex from the two eyes fire in conjunction with each other. No relevant growth factors have yet been found. Rearing in the dark appears to extend the duration of the critical period. Any overall theory about mechanisms that determine the beginning and end of the critical period will have to account for the fact that there are different critical periods for different parts of the system. Almost certainly multiple mechanisms are involved.

In summary, the area of visual deprivation is a very active area of research at the moment because there are some well-defined behavioral observations that can be correlated with anatomical and physiological effects. The results are important for general theories about the development of the nervous system as well as for clinically important deficits in humans.

Further reading

Hubel DH, Wiesel TN, Le Vay S (1977): Plasticity of ocular dominance columns in monkey striate cortex. *Phil Trans R Soc Lond B* 278:377–409

Movshon JA, Van Sluyters RC (1981): Visual neural development. *Ann Rev Psychol* 32:477–522

Sherman SM, Spear PD (1982): Organization of the visual pathways in normal and visually deprived cats. *Physiol Rev* 62:738–855

Wiesel TN (1982): Postnatal development of the visual cortex and the influence of environment. *Nature* 299:583–591

Vision, Extrageniculostriate

Tauba Pasik and Pedro Pasik

The visual system of mammals comprises three major interconnected neuronal networks processing information at the retina, the thalamus (lateral geniculate nucleus), and the striate cortex. Destruction of the striate cortex entails the death of geniculate neurons projecting to that area (retrograde degeneration) and, in time, the death of some retinal ganglion cells as well (retrograde transneuronal degeneration). Certain visual functions are retained or recover, however, in the regions of the visual fields originally subserved by the destroyed areas. These functions are generically termed extrageniculostriate vision since they are carried out in the absence of the geniculostriate system. Such forms of vision have been studied in humans within areas of blindness in the visual field produced by cerebral lesions. Patients show homonymous field defects on standard visual field examination, but with special testing techniques, they may be able to localize targets within the perimetrically defined anopic area, as well as make judgments concerning the shape and predominant wavelength of the stimulus.

The main body of information on extrageniculostriate vision is gained from experimental studies in Old World monkeys where complete bilateral exclusion of the system can be accomplished surgically. These totally destriated monkeys provide data that circumvent the difficulties in interpretation derived from studies of function within restricted visual field defects, such as the possible effects of fixation shifts and of stray light. Results are validated only when histological examination verifies the completeness of the ablations. The responses of such animals to visual stimuli may be of the unlearned or learned types. The unlearned behaviors, which can be elicited from the early postoperative period, include the pupillary light reflex, the blink to a sudden increase in illumination, the visual pursuit of large bright targets, and the optokinetic and flicker-induced nystagmi. Although present, these functions are not altogether normal. The blink response requires a considerably higher stimulus intensity. Optokinetic nystagmus can be evoked only at low stimulus velocities, and its peak frequency is lower than in the intact animal.

Learned responses require a certain amount of training to become manifest. Thus, destriated monkeys can be taught to reach accurately for targets as small as 1.5 degrees of visual angle, even when the exposure duration is below the threshold for visually elicited saccadic eye movements. This condition rules out the possible role of proprioceptive clues, which could result from directing the eyes toward the target. The earlier notion that these animals react like a photocell, i.e., to fluctuations in the total amount of luminous flux entering the eyes, has been superseded by the demonstration that they can learn to discriminate stimuli equated for this dimension but that differed in brightness (as given by the luminance), area, and contour, or only in brightness and area. They can also succeed through prolonged training to distinguish a circle from a triangle of equal area and brightness and, therefore, of the same

flux. Differences in the amount of contour are not critical for success. Finally there is also a residual capacity to utilize wavelength clues to solve a problem (Fig. 1). The last function may be mediated by the rod system since the spectral sensitivity curves of these monkeys determined at photopic levels are shifted toward scotopic values, implying an absence of information processing by the cone system.

The residual capacity to discriminate patterns may depend, as has been proposed for the normal, on the ability to process certain types of information contained in the figures, such as

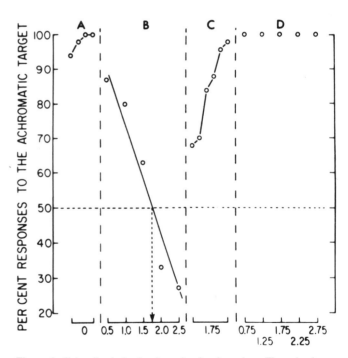

Figure 1. Color discrimination by a destriated monkey. The animal was rewarded after selection of an achromatic target presented together with a red target. The horizontal scales represent the log density of neutral filters added to the achromatic target, except that zero indicates no filters added. A. Learning profile of a monkey following the ablations. B. Performance dropped progressively in critical trials (both targets rewarded) with decreasing luminance of the achromatic figure, and eventually reversed, i.e., the monkey selected the red target more often than the achromatic stimulus. By intrapolation it was estimated that the equal brightness level for the two stimuli (50% responses to each) could be achieved by adding a 1.75 ND filter to the achromatic target. C. Learning profile with the targets behaviorally matched for brightness. D. Performance was maintained on critical trials despite increasing or decreasing the luminance of the achromatic stimulus. From Pasik and Pasik (1980).

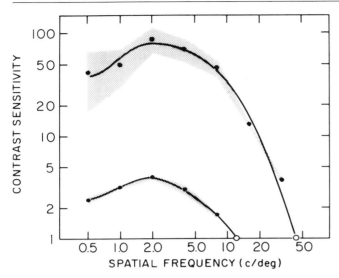

Figure 2. Contrast sensitivity functions of normal (top curve) and destriated monkeys (bottom curve). Each solid circle represents the group mean ($N = 4$), and the shaded area is the extent of the standard deviation. Open symbols indicate the extrapolated high-frequency cutoff points. The solid curves are the best-fitting lines determined by exponential equations for the high and low frequency limbs. From Pasik and Pasik (1980).

the inherent spatial frequency components, and their contrasts and orientations. In fact, it has been found that destriated monkeys not only can solve a vertical versus horizontal luminous bar problem, but are able to distinguish a vertical bar from another deviating only 7–8 degrees from the vertical. This threshold represents a drop in sensitivity of about 18 dB with respect to the values obtained from normal monkeys (1.2–1.6 degrees). Such preparation can discriminate sinusoidal gratings of high contrast (79%) but of spatial frequencies between 0.5 and 10 cycles per degree. When contrast thresholds are obtained at these spatial frequencies, a contrast sensitivity function emerges (Fig. 2) with the peak sensitivity occurring as in normal monkeys at about 2 cycles per degree. The sensitivity values, however, are much lower, corresponding to a loss of approximately 27 dB. The theoretical high spatial frequency cutoff, representing the highest frequency discernible at maximum contrast, has been considered a measure of visual acuity. The value obtained in destriated monkeys is about 12 cycles per degree, equivalent to a visual acuity of 2.5 minutes of arc, in turn a level no worse than 20/80 on the Snellen chart (acuity of normal monkeys: 0.7 minutes of arc).

The various expressions of extrageniculostriate vision must depend on neuronal networks that receive information from the retina via sites of termination of retinal fibers other than the lateral geniculate nucleus. The question of critical structures in the remaining brain that mediate these functions is explored by testing destriated monkeys after additional lesions.

Studies of this kind have ruled out the importance of both the isocortical (inferotemporal region) and allocortical (parahippocampal and retrosplenial) segments of the temporal cortex.

Ablations of the superior colliculi in destriated monkeys abolish space localization as well as the ability to discriminate between figures equated for total luminous flux. Similarly, the latter capacity does not recover when, instead of the tectum, the lesions destroy the inferior pulvinar nuclei, or when the striate cortex removal is extended to include the circumstriate cortex. Medial pretectal lesions and/or midsagittal section of the posterior commissure interfere with pupillary function (incomplete constriction to light), and eliminate the blink reflex to increased illumination. All of these lesions fail, however, to completely eliminate the recovery of the ability to distinguish between targets differing in flux, and to react with nystagmus to successive stimuli traversing the visual field (optokinetic nystagmus). These functions are abolished only by additional discrete bilateral lesions of the accessory optic system at the surface of the mesodiencephalic junction. It appears that this system is extremely sensitive to flux differences since the functions can still be carried out after midsagittal section of the optic chiasm which preserves only the minor uncrossed component. It is important to note that restricted lesions of most of these structures in otherwise normal monkeys, i.e., with intact striate cortex, produce no gross impairments of the functions studied, except for the pupillary reactions after pretectal damage.

This discussion leads to the conclusion that the striate cortex plays a preeminent role in most of the investigated functions since its total excision results in an initial failure of these capacities. The functional recovery that occurs in time, and that may involve prolonged training, suggests a process of reorganization in remaining structures that contribute only subtly to the behavior of the normal subject. Although studies to date point to collicular-pulvinar-circumstriate cortex networks for the recovery of the more elaborate forms of behavior, and to the accessory optic system for the probably basic distinction of total luminous flux differences, close to nothing is known of the possible participation of other structures where retinal fibers terminate, namely, some discrete pretectal nuclei, as well as the suprachiasmatic and pregeniculate nuclei.

Further reading

Campion J, Latto R, Smith YM (1983): Is blindsight an effect of scattered light, spared cortex, and near-threshold vision? (with Open Peer Commentaries). *Behav Brain Sci* 6:423–486

Keating EG, Dineen J (1982): Visual-motor transforms of the primate tectum. In: *Advances in the Analysis of Visual Behavior,* Ingle DJ, Goodale MA, Mansfield RJW, eds. Cambridge: MIT Press

Pasik T, Pasik P (1980): Extrageniculostriate vision in primates. In: *Neuroophthalmology,* Lessel S, van Dalen JTW, eds. Amsterdam: Excerpta Medica

Pasik P, Pasik T (1982): Visual functions in monkeys after total removal of visual cerebral cortex. In: *Contributions to Sensory Physiology,* Vol 7, Neff WD, ed. New York: Academic Press

Vision, Visual Cortex, and Frequency Analysis

Daniel A. Pollen and James P. Gaska

D.H. Hubel and T.N. Wiesel opened the modern era of visual cortical physiology with their paper on the receptive field properties of simple and complex cells in the visual cortex of the cat. Both cell types are selectively responsive to the orientation of an elongated slit of light. These neurons may be sensitive either to one or both directions of movement perpendicular to the preferred orientation. Neurons with different orientation preferences are anatomically segregated within columns or sheets that are further interspersed within ocular dominance columns.

Frequency analysis has been used both to test the extent of linear processing by visual neurons and to provide an estimate of their spatial frequency selectivity. Sine-wave gratings, that is, gratings with luminance modulated sinusoidally along one dimension, are either drifted or counterphased across a neuron's receptive field. The majority of cortical neurons exhibit bandpass spatial frequency tuning curves, that is, they are sensitive to a particular spatial frequency and much less so to spatial frequencies higher or lower. The range of peak spatial frequencies of different cells with receptive fields located near the fovea in the monkey may cover up to 6 octaves, and the full band width at half amplitude may range from just under 1 octave to a little over 2 octaves with mean values of about 1.5 octaves. Electrophysiological observations on cortical neurons are generally consonant with the results of a wealth of psychophysical studies on spatial frequency selective channels that have followed the pioneer studies of FW Campbell and JG Robson.

Simple and complex cell types

The receptive fields of simple cells along their width dimensions are defined by their pure on or off responses to stationary flashed stimuli. The excitatory and inhibitory zones are mutually antagonistic. The receptive fields often consist of two or three alternating bands of excitatory and inhibitory zones, although fields with additional weak side lobes are also found. Simple cells have been shown to have approximately linear spatial summation across the width of their receptive fields. The periodicity of the excitatory and inhibitory subfields, the essentially balanced antagonism of the excitatory and inhibitory subfields, and the approximately linear spatial summation of simple cells are responsible for the bandpass type of spatial frequency selectivity of the neurons. Smaller spacing between subfields will lead to selectivity for higher spatial frequencies, and an increase in the number of subfields will produce narrower spatial frequency bandwidths.

Although the preferred spatial frequencies and bandwidths of complex cells span essentially the same range as those for simple cells, the nonlinear spatial summation properties of complex cells make the mechanisms that produce spatial frequency selectivity much less apparent. Complex cells respond to stationary flashed slits of light with both an on and off response at most positions across the receptive field width, although there may be small regions at the flanks of the receptive field which give pure on or off responses. Whereas the response of simple cells to drifting sine wave gratings consists of a truncated sine wave response pattern (the truncation is due to a low or zero rate of spontaneous activity of simple cells and their inability to signal negative response rates), the response to complex cells to a drifting grating are characterized by an increase in the mean firing rate above and below which a smaller modulated component may sometimes be superimposed. Studies of the receptive fields of complex cells have shown that they may be composed of linearly summating subunits that are rectified before being summed. The subunits have properties similar to simple cells and account for the spatial frequency tuning properties of complex cells.

Gabor functions

S. Marcelja has shown that the one-dimensional receptive field profiles of simple cells can be closely approximated by the product of a Gaussian and a sinusoid or co-sinusoid. These field profiles resemble the elementary signals that Dennis Gabor described in the time-temporal frequency domains in the mid-1940s. Here Gabor functions are centered at a given position and spatial frequency and provide for the simultaneous optimal localization of a signal in both the spatial and spatial frequency domains. Therefore, to the extent that the receptive field profiles and spatial frequency selectivity curves of simple cells resemble, respectively, those of Gabor elemental signals and their frequency transforms, the analysis of the retinal image by simple cells is the finest grain sampling that a filter set can achieve simultaneously for spatial position and spatial frequency.

Phase information is preserved when the even and odd symmetrical pair members have a common axis of symmetry; that is, the responses of a pair of neurons to drifting sine wave gratings would be 90° apart. The field profiles of many simple cells are not precisely purely even-symmetrical or purely odd-symmetrical. These phase lags do not present a theoretical problem as long as the relative phase offset between pair members is close to 90°, as has been demonstrated experimentally. Pairs of odd symmetrical simple cells with 180° phase offsets, required to preserve information that would otherwise be lost due to response truncation, have also been shown experimentally. Thus, if the four basic types of simple cells (Fig. 1) are present at each retinal position (x,y), for each spatial frequency and orientation, and if the information space is sampled with sufficient density to meet the requirements of Shannon's sampling theorem, then the information present at the simple cell stage may provide a complete representation of the information contained in the retinal image. There is no necessity

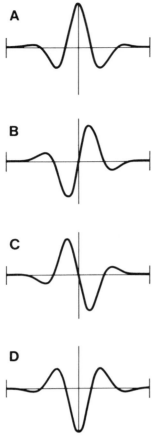

Figure 1. Four elementary one-dimensional Gabor signals sharing a common axis of symmetry are shown. The "on-center" even-symmetrical function $e^{-1/2(x/\alpha)^2} \cos 2\pi f_o x$ is shown in A; the odd-symmetrical functions $e^{-1/2(x/\alpha)^2} \sin 2\pi f_o x$ and $-e^{-1/2(x/\alpha)^2} \sin 2\pi f_o x$ are shown in B and C, and the "off-center" even-symmetrical function $-e^{-/2(x/\alpha)^2} \cos 2\pi f_o x$ is shown in D. The value of f_o is 2.8 c/deg., α is 0.137 deg.; the extent of the horizontal axis is 1°, and the full bandwidth at half-amplitude of the Fourier transform of these functions is, in all cases, 1.54 octaves. From Pollen DA, Foster KH, Gaska JP (1985): Phase-dependent response characteristics of visual cortical neurons. In: *Models of the Visual Cortex*. Rose D, Dobson VG, ed. Sussex: John Wiley and Sons. Reprinted by permission of John Wiley and Sons, Ltd.

artificial intelligence community, have not been shown to be applicable to these early stages of visual processing.

Although the Gabor function is a very good approximation to the simple cell receptive field, other functions have been proposed. Richard Young suggests that simple cells could be built up from an operation taking successive DOOGs (difference of off-set Gaussians). Each Gaussian represents either the excitatory or inhibitory envelope generated from a cell at the preceding level of processing. Successive differences would be used to build up neurons with increasing numbers of side lobes and correspondingly higher spatial frequencies and narrower spatial frequency band widths. These field profiles would closely resemble successive orders of Gaussian derivatives that may make up a complete set. The very slight differences between profiles made up from DOOGs and either the Gabor functions or Gaussian derivatives are so small that the experimental evidence has not yet resolved which model provides the best fit to simple cell receptive fields. All three sets of functions have the property of giving a close-to-ideal approximation for the simultaneous localization of a signal in both the spatial frequency and spatial domain.

Simple cells can be said to extract a spatially localized spatial frequency component with preservation of both spatial frequency and phase information at a given spatial position. At the complex cell stage a spatial frequency amplitude may be represented, but it is not yet clear whether phase information can be retained at this stage. Little is known about how information from simple and complex cells is used at still higher cortical levels.

Further reading

Primary sources
Campbell FW, Robson JG (1968): Application of Fourier analysis to the visibility of gratings. *J Physiol* 197:551–566
Foster KH, Gaska JP, Nagler M, Pollen DA (1985): Spatial and temporal frequency selectivity of neurones in visual cortical areas V1 and V2 of the macaque monkey. *J Physiol* 365:331–363.
Hubel DH, Wiesel TN (1962): Receptive fields, binocular interaction and functional architecture in the cat's visual cortex. *J Physiol* 160:106–154
Marcelja S (1980): Mathematical description of the responses of simple cortical cells. *J Opt Soc Am* 70:1297–1300
Movshon JA, Thompson ID, Tolhurst DV (1978): Receptive field organization of complex cells in the cat's striate cortex. *J Physiol* 283:79–99
Pollen DA, Ronner SF (1981): Phase relationship between adjacent cells in the visual cortex of the cat. *Science* 212:1409–1411

Review
Pollen DA, Ronner SF (1983): Visual cortical neurons as localized spatial frequency filters. *IEEE Trans Sys Man Cybernet* SMC-13:907–916

at the level of the simple cell stage to resort to models that retain only line or edge information since contrast gradation may be retained within the ensemble of simple cell activity. Laplacian zero crossing models, which are of interest to the

Visual Adaptation, Dark, Light

John C. Armington

The visual system works effectively over an enormous range of light intensities. This is made possible by its remarkable ability to adjust its operating level to match the ambient illumination, an ability that is called adaptation. Dark adaptation is the process of adjusting to total darkness or to lower levels of illumination; light adaptation is the reverse. The study of adaptation is important for a variety of practical reasons as well as for an understanding of basic visual function. The most detailed knowledge of adaptational processes has come from psychophysics, but the results have always been pertinent to physiological theory and experimentation.

Adaptation is mediated by a combination of actions. The pupil, which opens with the ambient level of illumination, is one of these. In the human, the pupil can control the light reaching the retina by a factor of only about 10, an amount that can account for only a small part of the entire adaptive range. In some species, such as those having slit pupils, a much greater range is available. In other species, but not humans, there is a migration of screening pigment at the rear of the retina and of the rod receptors themselves so as to shield them when the eye is exposed to high levels of illumination. The main mechanisms of adaptation, however, lie within the receptors and the neural structures of the retina.

The human retina, as that of many species, is duplex. It possesses a photopic or cone system that works at high levels of illumination and a scotopic or rod system that works at low. Thus, the large range of adaptation seen in the human eye is achieved by a change from one system to the other as well as by adjustments of sensitivity within the individual systems. A classic way of describing these changes is in terms of a dark adaptation curve (Fig. 1).

Such a curve is obtained by first exposing the eye to bright light and then placing it in total darkness. The threshold to a brief test flash is determined at intervals as dark adaptation progresses, and the results are plotted as shown.

The dark adaptation curve has two limbs. During the very first minutes of darkness, the threshold drops rapidly and then tapers off to a plateau. After a few more minutes, the curve drops rapidly a second time and approaches a lower plateau. As many as 45 minutes may be required to reach the final level, the so-called absolute threshold. A large body of evidence shows that the first limb describes an increase or recovery of photopic sensitivity in the dark and the second, one of scotopic sensitivity. A change in the relative spectral sensitivity, i.e., the sensitivity of the eye to different wavelengths of light, is an important part of this evidence. When measured at the time of the lower plateau of the dark adaptation curve, spectral sensitivity is found to be greatest near 500 nm and matches that of rhodopsin, the photosensitive pigment found in the rods. When it is measured at the time of the first plateau, the relative sensitivity curve maximizes near 555 nm, as is characteristic of the photopic system. This change in relative sensitivity is known as the Purkinje shift, and the transition from the first limb to the second limb of the dark adaptation curve that accompanies the shift is known as the rod-cone break. Stimuli above the break appear colored; those below, colorless.

The form of the dark adaptation changes in a predictable manner with the stimulus conditions. Figure 1 is typical of the one produced by a blue stimulus delivered to a peripheral retinal position where both rods and cones are numerous. When the dark adaptation curve is measured with red test stimuli or with stimuli restricted to the rod-free foveal region, there is only a photopic limb as indicated by the dashed line. A lower threshold is measured with a stimulus of relatively large area than small. If the period of light adaptation that precedes dark adaptation is not extended in time, but lasts 2 or 3 minutes or less, dark adaptation progresses substantially more rapidly than indicated in Figure 1. Finally, it should be noted that there is a trade-off between visual sensitivity and resolution during dark adaptation. Under conditions of high sensitivity, acuity is low.

Since visual stimulation begins with the bleaching of photopigment within the receptors, it is obvious that light-adapted rods will contain less unbleached rhodopsin than dark-adapted ones. At one time it was postulated that the visual threshold during dark adaptation is directly related to the concentration of this photopigment in the receptors. Techniques have now been developed that make it possible to measure rhodopsin in the living eye during dark adaptation. These disprove the simple photochemical hypothesis by showing that the logarithm

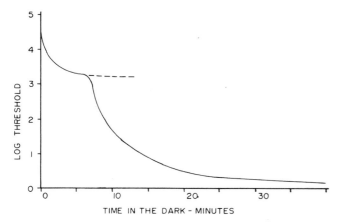

Figure 1. Dark adaptation curve. The solid line is a plot of threshold (inarbitrary units) against the length of time the eye has been in darkness. The dashed line is an extrapolation of the upper or photopic limb of the curve. The lower limb is scotopic.

of the visual threshold is approximately proportional to the amount of rhodopsin bleached. Important events may take place during adaptation in intracellular transmission as well as in the synaptic transmission in the retina.

Light adaptation

Technical problems render it difficult to measure the temporal course of the threshold increase that follows the onset of light adaptation in a manner parallel to that of the dark adaptation curve. Although there is no method that is strictly analogous, thresholds can be measured to flashes of light presented at some short fixed interval of dark adaptation after light adaptations of differing length. Results of this kind of experiment show that light adaptation proceeds rapidly at first, and then more slowly. Under some conditions change can be seen as much as 30 minutes after the onset of light adaptation. A problem with this type of measurement, however, is that the degree of light adaptation influences the subsequent rate of dark adaptation, so that two variables are confounded in the result.

A more straightforward measure is provided by the incremental threshold, the threshold for detecting a flash of light against a steady lighted background. Some typical results are shown in Figure 2.

Figure 2A shows a plot of the incremental threshold as dependent on the luminance of the background. At low levels, the background has no effect, but as the background is raised the threshold rises, at first gradually and then more rapidly. At higher levels there is a second plateau followed by a second

rise. As in dark adaptation curves, the two limbs of the plot can be attributed to the participation of the rod and cone systems. When the eye is adapted to low levels, the rod system is most sensitive, but at higher adaptations scotopic sensitivity drops below that of the cones.

Also, as in the case of the dark adaptation curve, the limbs of the increment threshold versus adaptation curve depend on the testing conditions such as the size of the stimuli, their location on the retina, and their spectral composition. The example just examined is typical of orange yellow stimuli presented against a blue green background in the parafoveal region. Other conditions result in a less conspicuous separation of the two retinal systems. A blue stimulus, which favors the scotopic system, presented against a red adaptation, which is effective in reducing the sensitivity of the photopic system, can produce an increment threshold curve in which the scotopic function is completely uncovered, as shown in Figure 2B. Different sectors of this curve may be distinguished for theoretical as well as descriptive purposes. Throughout the middle of the range (b), the curve is nearly linear and hence, approximates the classic Weber's law. At the upper end (a), the curve swings steeply upward to become nearly vertical. This is known as the saturation region. At the lower end the curve bends (c) and becomes horizontal (d), thus marking the region where the background is too weak to have effect. Several theoretical accounts of the incremental threshold curve have invoked the concept of an intrinsic activity or noise within the receptor systems that combines with the excitation produced by the background to raise the threshold. In the same vein, dark adaptation and incremental threshold curves have

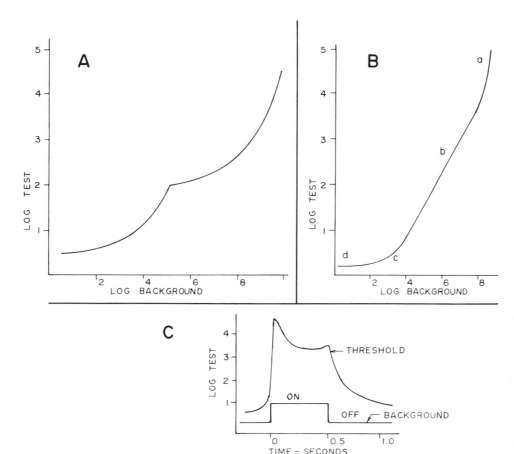

Figure 2. Incremental threshold curves. A. The threshold is plotted against the intensity of the background stimulus. The lower branch describes the sensitivity of the scotopic system; the upper that of the photopic. B. This curve was obtained under conditions where scotopic sensitivity could be followed over a wide range. The sectors are identified in the text. C. Incremental threshold as measured against a slowly flashing background. The time that the background is on is indicated. All threshold and background intensities in this figure are expressed in arbitrary units.

been related to one another with some success by postulating a dark light, an intrinsic excitation that persists after light adaptation. Although it does not give rise to visual sensation, dark light acts as a background against which the test flash must be seen during dark adaptation.

The procedures of light and dark adaptation are useful for investigating color processes. If, for example, incremental thresholds are measured with monochromatic test flashes presented against monochromatic backgrounds, the photopic sector shown in Figure 2A may break up, depending upon the particular wavelengths used, into two or more constituent limbs. By measuring the incremental threshold function systematically for a wide range of test and adaptation wavelengths, it is possible to determine the spectral sensitivities of these limbs and thus, to define the color processes they represent. Color information may also be gained from the dark adaptation curve if it is measured with monochromatic test stimuli following preexposure to monochromatic fields.

Rapid adaptational changes

The initial changes in visual sensitivity, those that accompany the very onset of light and dark adaptation, are also of considerable interest. These have been measured by superimposing a small, brief test flash upon a larger adaptation field that is switched on and off periodically. The timing between the test flash and the adaptation light is under experimental control. The threshold measured when the adaptation background is on an incremental threshold while that measured with it off is not. This type of experiment, therefore, helps to define the transition from one type of threshold measure to another. The experiment, as shown in Figure 2C, indicates that the threshold to the flash begins to rise shortly before the onset of the adaptation light. It reaches a maximum near the time of adaptation onset, drops somewhat, and then climbs to a

second, but lower maximum at the time of offset. Sensitivity then gradually returns. The fact that the threshold starts to rise before the onset of the adaptation stimulus has been attributed to the speed with which information travels through the visual system. The relatively weak test flash gives rise to signals that travel more slowly to the level of the visual system where the threshold decision is made than do those of the stronger adaptation stimulus.

Electrophysiological evidence

The phenomena of dark and light adaptation have been investigated electrophysiologically both with the electroretinogram in the human subject and also with unit recording in other species. These potentials show a progressive increase in sensitivity that advances with dark adaptation. The changes seen with light and dark adaptation are similar to those seen psychophysically, but exact comparisons can seldom be made because it is difficult to conduct psychophysics and electrophysiology under strictly comparable conditions. Nevertheless, electrophysical experiments have helped to clarify the understanding of the adaptation process. They are also useful because they provide information regarding the visual process away from the threshold conditions to which psychophysics is limited.

Further reading

Barlow HB (1972): Dark and light adaptation: Psychophysics. In: *Handbook of Sensory Physiology,* VII/4, Jameson D, Hurvich LM, eds. New York: Springer-Verlag

Bartlett NR (1965): Dark adaptation and light adaptation. In: *Vision and Visual Perception.* Graham CH, ed. New York: Wiley

Rushton WAH (1981): Visual adaptation. In: *Adler's Physiology of the Eye: Clinical Application,* 7th ed, Moses, RA, ed. St Louis: Mosby

Wyszecki G, Stiles WS (1982): *Color Science, Concepts and Methods, Quantatative Data and Formulas,* 2nd ed. New York: Wiley

Visual Aftereffects

Jeremy M. Wolfe

Exposure to visual stimuli can alter the detectability and appearance of subsequent stimuli. These aftereffects fall into three broad classes:

1. Retinal effects (afterimages)
2. Central effects due to fatigue
3. Central effects not entirely due to fatigue

Aftereffects are important not so much for their impact on normal vision but for the information they reveal about structure and function in human vision. Aftereffects are among the most powerful tools in the noninvasive dissection of the human visual system.

Retinal effects

The first step in the transduction of light into electrochemical signals in the nervous system is the bleaching of photopigment in photoreceptors (the rods and cones) of the eye. Once bleached, photopigment must return to its unbleached state before it can participate again in the detection of light. If a substantial proportion of photopigment is bleached, visual sensitivity will be reduced. On a sunny day, a high proportion of the photopigment may be bleached. If one then enters a dimly lit room, it may be hard to see until some of the photopigment has returned to its unbleached state. In this example, the entire retina has been exposed to bright light. Suppose that a restricted region is exposed (e.g., by a camera flash) and bleached. The corresponding location in the visual field will be less sensitive to light. If you look at a white wall, the wall will appear darker in that part of the field. The dark spot is a simple negative afterimage, negative because the dark afterimage is the opposite of the bright inducing stimulus.

The afterimage is restricted to the stimulated part of the retina. Thus, it moves when the eyes move. Its size is described by the visual angle subtended by the inducing stimulus. As a result, the afterimage looks larger if viewed on a distant surface (e.g., the far wall) and smaller if viewed on a close surface (e.g., the far wall) and smaller if viewed on a close surface (Emmert's law). Stimuli that are stable on the retina fade from view after a few seconds. Normally, small eye movements keep images in constant motion. Afterimages will move with the eyes and so are always stabilized. Unless the background changes (e.g., by blinking), an afterimage will fade after a few seconds.

Color vision is made possible by the existence of three different cone photopigments. Each has a different sensitivity to light of different wavelengths. A colored light will effect the cone pigments differently. A red light, for example, will selectively reduce the sensitivity of the long wavelength cone. As a result, a white stimulus that activated all cones roughly equally now will activate short- and medium-wavelength cones more than the long cones, creating a bluish green aftereffect. In general, exposure to a colored light will cause a white light to take on the complementary color.

A very bright flash of light will give rise to a positive afterimage that will glow in the dark for some time. A positive afterimage is a persistent copy of the original stimulus. It is analogous to the persistent sensation felt after the skin is slapped. Different color mechanisms recover at different rates. As a result, the positive afterimage often will change color, going through a series of very saturated hues before vanishing (often referred to as a "flight of colors").

Afterimages, both positive and negative, are not entirely explained by the bleaching and recovery of photopigments in the photoreceptors or even by neural events restricted to the retina. Nevertheless, a photoreceptor-based explanation gives a fair picture of standard afterimage phenomena.

Central effects due to fatigue

As light reduces sensitivity to light, so other stimuli can reduce sensitivity more specifically. For example, since the 1960s, one of the standard stimuli used in studying human vision has been the sinusoidal grating. Such a grating looks like a set of parallel, out-of-focus bars. Its luminance profile is sinusoidal. Different spatial frequencies are created by making the bars fatter (low frequency) or finer (high frequency). For a variety of reasons, such stimuli are the preferred way to study the visual system's sensitivity to different sizes. Exposure (or adaptation) to a grating will reduce sensitivity to other gratings of that and nearby spatial frequencies. An adapting grating of low spatial frequency will have no influence on the visibility of high-frequency gratings, and vice versa. Further, vertical gratings will not influence the visibility of horizontal gratings. The selectivity of adaptation is due to selective fatigue of mechanisms tuned for a specific orientation. Similar aftereffects of exposure to motion and depth exist.

These aftereffects tell us about the early stages of visual processing. There are no "cow" or "Chevy" aftereffects. The visual system analyzes its input for certain basic features and only adaptation to those features or their simple combinations gives rise to aftereffects. These aftereffects show interocular transfer. If the adapting stimulus is shown to one eye, the aftereffect can be measured with the other eye. Since information from the two eyes is not combined until it reaches the visual cortex, the physical site of adaptation cannot be prior to cortex. Variations on the interocular transfer experiment can reveal much about the structure of the monocular and binocular pathways in human vision. Even though they do not occur in the retina, the aftereffects still are restricted to the part of the visual field that was stimulated, another indication of low-level processing.

Central effects not entirely due to fatigue

An example from the third class of aftereffects has been produced by rivers (Aristotle), military parades (Purkinje, 1825), and waterfalls (Addams, 1842). Taking the last case, if one looks at water pouring down a fall, stationary objects on the shore subsequently may appear to drift uphill (motion aftereffect). A characteristic of such aftereffects is that exposure to one stimulus alters the appearance of another. Aftereffects of this sort also exist for tilt, depth, and various combinations of basic stimulus dimensions. The most famous combination is the McCollough effect. If one views black and green vertical stripes, and black and red horizontal stripes, subsequently viewed black and white stripes will look pink if vertical and greenish if horizontal. The color of the aftereffect is contingent on the orientation of the stripes.

These aftereffects often have been explained as by-products of fatigue just as colored negative afterimages are explained as by-products of photoreceptor bleaching. In the case of the waterfall, motion down would fatigue downward motion detectors. A stationary stimulus now would stimulate upward detectors more than downward and would appear to drift upward. There are a variety of reasons for doubting this explanation. The most compelling is the duration of aftereffects in the third class. Fatigue aftereffects of the second class last for seconds or minutes. Class three aftereffects can last for hours, days, weeks, or even months, as in the case of the McCollough effect. This means that the aftereffects long outlast any measurable fatigue.

Aftereffects of this class involve changes in the definitions of visual quantities that are not fixed in the retinal image. For example, with the eye continually in motion, there is no such thing as a physically stationary stimulus. The motion aftereffect may be the visual system's way of fine-tuning its definition of stationary. The third class of aftereffects actually may be a very simple form of learning or memory.

Class three aftereffects are restricted to the stimulated part of the visual field and, with the puzzling exception of those involving color (e.g., McCollough), show interocular transfer.

Further reading

Class one
Brown JL (1965): Afterimages. In: *Vision and Visual Perception.* CH Graham, ed. New York: Wiley

Class two and three
Favreau OE (1976): Negative aftereffects in visual processes. *Sci Am* 235:42–48

On the uses of aftereffects
Wolfe JM (1983): Hidden visual processes. *Sci Am* 248:94–103

Visual Cortex

Max Cynader

The word cortex means "bark" in Latin, highlighting the fact that the cortex is a folded sheet of tissue, with a constant thickness near 2 mm, wrapped around the cereberal hemispheres. The cortex as a whole has expanded enormously in phylogeny, and the part of the cortex dealing with vision has participated in this expansion. In primates, the term visual cortex refers to the area called V1 by physiologists, and area 17 or striate cortex by anatomists. It receives its major input from the eyes via a relay in the lateral geniculate nucleus of the thalamus. Recent physiological mapping experiments have greatly expanded our knowledge of other cortical areas, outside the primary visual cortex, that are also concerned with processing visual information. There are over a dozen distinct visual cortical areas, each with its own representation of visual space, which together cover as much as 50% of the cortical surface. The function of these extrastriate cortical areas remains uncertain, but accumulating evidence assigns different areas special roles in tasks like motion perception, depth perception, color vision, control of eye and limb movement, object recognition, and visual attention. There is evidence for two streams of cortical processing areas, both originating in V1, one stream concerned primarily with recognition and identification, the other with attention and localization. The primary visual cortex can be thought of as a funnel in these processing streams through which all input must pass before it can be further analyzed.

The structure and function of the striate cortex are best evaluated within the context of its location at the confluence of these processing streams and the requirements of the image processing problems to which the cortex is the solution. Since the visual cortex must provide appropriate outputs to the multiple visual areas with which it is connected, it must convey information about several different aspects of the stimulus simultaneously. It must localize objects and their borders accurately, and it must operate on the visual image simultaneously at several different spatial scales. This last requirement arises not only because objects and textures of interest come in different shapes and sizes, but also because the combined signal from elements operating at different spatial scales enables us to identify and localize discontinuities (an oriented edge, for instance) with greater certainty and precision than would be possible with elements operating at only one spatial scale.

Microelectrode recordings, measuring the activity of individual visual cortical cells while an animal is shown a variety of visual stimuli, were pioneered by D. Hubel and T. Wiesel. They and more recent workers have shown that cortical units are differentially active depending on the orientation, length, width, contrast, and color of the stimulus. Stimulus location, (including location in depth) and speed and direction of motion in both two- and three-dimensional space can also profoundly influence cortical cell activity. The evidence that activity of individual cortical cells can be altered in response to several different aspects of the visual stimulus has complicated early notions of striate cells as feature detectors or analyzers. If cells are indeed feature analyzers, then they must be carrying on several different analyses in parallel. More recent formulations emphasize the functions of single units within the broader context of the pattern analysis problems to be solved. The requirement that information be transmitted about a variety of stimulus parameters simultaneously and that this information be available at several spatial scales imposes some severe design constraints on visual cortical architecture. Several parameters of the organization of the visual cortex may reflect the task of simultaneously receiving, representing, and distributing information about multiple facets of the external world. These include columnar and surface organization, laminar organization, and chemical specificity.

Columnar and surface organization

The microelectrode studies of Hubel and Wiesel were the first to reveal common properties among cortical cells running from surface to white matter in the same region of the cortex. First among these commonalities to be discovered was a tendency for neurons encountered in a given penetration perpendicular to the cortical surface to show the same preferred stimulus orientation. In oblique penetrations, there is a progressive shift in preferred stimulus orientation as the electrode is advanced. A second columnar property is preferred eye input. On a given perpendicular penetration, neurons not only share the same preferred orientation, but also respond best to stimuli presented via a given eye. Several other cortical response properties may display columnar organization, but the evidence is not always as strong as that for orientation and ocular preference. These include direction selectivity, spatial frequency selectivity, motion in depth selectivity, and color specificity. Recent interest has focused not only on the columnar organization of cortical neurons, but also on the tangential layout of these columns. This has been approached either by making many repeated electrode penetrations into the cortex and assaying response properties at each location, or by the use of anatomical methods. The method of transneuronal autoradiography is one of several which has been used to visualize the tangential distribution of ocular dominance columns in Old World monkeys. Figure 1, shows that in a tangential view of the cortex of rhesus monkey, these regions take the form of elongated bands running across the surface. The center-to-center spacing between neighboring eye dominance bands is about 0.4 mm. Other approaches using the 2-deoxyglucose method and voltage-sensitive dyes have been used to visualize the tangential distribution of other putative columnar systems, including those for spatial frequency, color, depth, and orientation. The relationship among the different columnar systems is under investigation.

Figure 1. The distribution of inputs representing the two eyes in the visual cortex of *Macaca fascicularis*. The figure is a montage produced from several sections through layer 4C of the cortex. One of the animal's eyes had been injected with ^{3}H-proline two weeks before perfusion, allowing for transport from the eye to the brightly striped areas of the photomicrograph. The stripes interdigitate with darker stripes representing inputs from the other eye. Scale bar, 5 mm. Reproduced with permission from Levay S, Connolly M, Houde J, Van Essen DC (1985): *J Neurosci* 5:486–501.

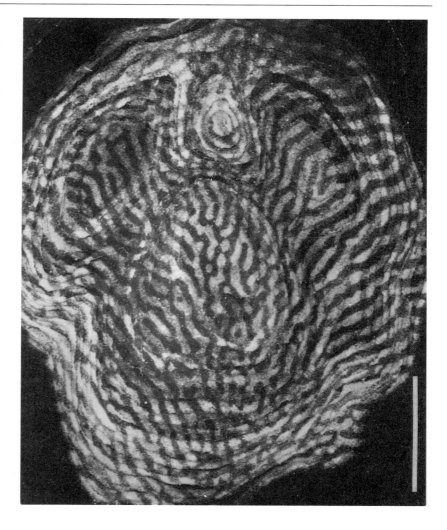

Figure 2. The tangential distribution of cytochrome oxidase activity in striate and prestriate cortex of squirrel monkey. The semicircular area on the right is striate cortex; the adjoining region, marked by the alternating light and dark bands is prestriate cortex. Note the distribution of cytochrome-oxidase rich blobs in striate cortex and the abrupt transition to a banded pattern at the striate-prestriate border. Calibration bar, 5 mm. Reproduced with permission from Tootell RB, Silverman MS, DeValois RL, Jacobs GH (1983): *Science* 220:737–739. Copyright 1983 by the AAAS.

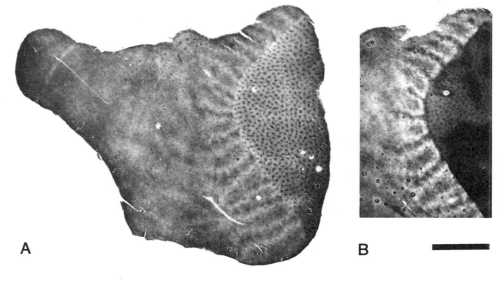

A

B

The chemistry of cortical columnar organization has taken a new turn with recent discoveries of a pattern of regularly repeating bloblike structures in primate striate cortex that stain heavily for the mitochondrial enzyme cytochrome oxidase. In tangential sections, the blobs are oval in shape, located in the center of ocular dominance bands in Old World monkeys, and elongated along the bands. In coronal sections, the blobs take the form of interrupted columns that are most clearly visible in layers 2 and 3 and less well defined in layers 4B, 5, and 6. These blobs can also be outlined with antibodies to glutamic acid decarboxylase (GAD), the synthetic enzyme for gamma-aminobutyric acid (GABA), a major inhibitory neurotransmitter within the cortex. Electron microscopic studies show an increased incidence of GAD-positive terminals within the blobs. The functional properties of cells within the blobs are distinguished from those outside these zones by showing strong tendencies for dominance by one eye or the other, by showing little or no orientation selectivity, and by responding in a highly selective fashion to colored stimuli, especially to chromatic borders. Figure 2 shows the cytochrome oxidase blobs as seen in tangential sections of the squirrel monkey striate cortex. It also shows that prestriate cortex contains bands of cells, running perpendicular to the striate-prestriate border, in which cytochrome oxidase activity is alternately elevated and depressed. Note the sharp transition between the bloblike arrays in striate cortex and the pattern of bands that occur in prestriate cortex. Microinjections of tracers within striate and prestriate cortex show that the striate blob regions connect preferentially to the thinner cytochrome-rich bands in prestriate cortex. The interblob regions of striate cortex connect to zones of reduced cytochrome activity in prestriate cortex.

Laminar organization

The cortex shows marked heterogeneity through its 2-mm thickness. Neurons in different layers have markedly different somal and dendritic shapes, packing densities, functional properties, and anatomical connections. The left-hand side of Figure 3 illustrates the lamination of the visual cortex as viewed with a cell body stain. An incomplete synopsis of some of the major connections of individual layers follows. Layer 6, the deepest layer of the striate cortex, projects back toward the lateral geniculate nucleus (LGN). Layer 5 projects heavily to the superior colliculus, a midbrain structure concerned with eye movements and visual attention. Layers 2 and 3 and parts of layer 4 send major outputs to other visual cortical areas. Layer 4C is the most important input layer, with subdivisions of this layer receiving inputs from specific layers of the LGN. LGN terminals, however, can also be found in layers 4A and in the cytochrome blobs of layer 3. Associated with the specificity of connections of different cortical layers is functional specificity. Units in layer 6 often respond best to extremely elongated stimuli, whereas neurons in the superficial layers (II and III) often prefer short bars. Neurons in layer 5 have the widest receptive fields of all cortical neurons and frequently respond well to spots of light as well as oriented bars. Binocular responses, dependent on the depth of the visual stimulus and on motion in depth, are generally most selective in layers II and III. Several circuit diagrams of cortical wiring have been proposed to show how information flows from the major input stage in layer 4C to other layers. These efforts are based on analysis of visual responses of cells in different layers, the study of anatomical interconnections between different layers, and on current source density analysis or measurement of unit responses following electrical stimulation or selective inactivation of afferent pathways. The models proposed thus far are

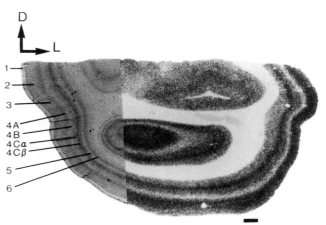

Figure 3. The laminar distribution of muscarinic acetycholine binding sites in *Macaca fascicularis* striate cortex, assessed using ^{3}H-quinuclindyl benzilate binding. The labeled side of this composite section is stained with cresyl violet for Nissl substance to reveal the cortical lamination. The right-hand side is a photograph of an autoradiogram in which increased optical density reflects greater numbers of receptors. Scale bar, 1 mm. Reproduced with permission from Shaw C, Cynader M (1986): *J Comp Neurol* 248:301–312.

suggestive and have heuristic value, but we are far from the goal of a full functional description of how information flows in the cortical circuit. What is clear, however, is that different layers of the cortex are specialized in their inputs, their outputs, and in their functional properties.

Chemical specificity

A recently discovered and striking feature of the cortex is its diversity of transmitter substances and receptors. Well over a dozen different substances are now thought to play a role in intercellular communication within striate cortex. Immunocytochemical methods have made it possible to identify populations of neurons, axons, and terminals containing particular neurotransmitters or neuromodulators within the cortex. The development of sensitive antibodies directed against norepinephrine, serotonin, acetylcholine, and their synthetic enzymes has enabled the identification of trajectories and, in some cases, the termination patterns of these fiber systems within the visual cortex. Thus, serotonergic fiber systems terminate extensively in layer 4 of the cortex, while noradrenergic fibers terminate most densely in layers V and VI. Antisera against vasoactive intestinal peptide (VIP), somatostatin, cholecystokinin, and their synthetic enzymes have revealed specific neuronal populations within the cortex containing these peptides. The peptide-containing neurons are usually nonpyramidal neurons with specific laminar distributions and morphological characteristics. The functional importance of many of these transmitters remains unknown although electrophysiological studies show that cholecystokinin or VIP application excites cortical neurons. In some instances peptides may be co-localized with other neurotransmitters in the same neurons. Many putative cholinergic neurons also stain positively for VIP; similarly many GABA-containing neurons in cat visual cortex contain somatostatin.

In parallel with immunocytochemical approaches to localize transmitters, studies of receptor populations within the visual cortex have provided evidence for precise organization of the receptors for these neurotransmitters. Using the new methods of in vitro receptor autoradiography, it has been possible to demonstrate specific laminar distributions for binding sites associated with amino acids (GABA, glutamate), monoamines (norepinepherine, serotonin), peptides (cholesystokinin, substance P), and other putative cortical neuromodulatory agents (acetylcholine, adenosine, and benzodiazepines). Each receptor population appears to display a specific and idiosyncratic laminar distribution. Figure 3 illustrates the laminar distribution of muscarinic acetylcholine receptors within striate cortex. Note the marked concentration of these receptors in layers 2, 3, 4a, and 4c with clear gaps in other layers. The laminar distributions of other transmitter binding sites show different patterns with concentrations in specific layers. The immunocytochemical and receptor binding studies summarized here support the notion that cortical processing mechanisms are compartmentalized and that different neurotransmitter systems operating in parallel may be handling different tasks. Additionally they show that the opportunity for multiple interactions among neuroactive substances and their receptors in the cortex is considerable. We still do not know why it is that so many different neurotransmitters and receptors exist within the cortex. One possibility is that they are part of the mechanisms that allow for multiplicity of function at varied temporal and spatial scales and for simultaneous representations of information regarding different stimulus parameters. Thus the association of GABA-related antibodies with the cytochrome oxidase blobs may reflect a particular association between this neurotransmitter system and color vision mechanisms. There is in fact, good evidence that different neurotransmitters and also different receptor subtypes may operate at a variety of time scales. Similarly the spatial precision of different chemically defined systems within the cortex varies. For example, individual noradrenergic fibers distribute in a very diffuse pattern across the cortical surface while VIP neurons are sharply confined in their distribution. Both transmitters cause increases in cyclic adenosine monophosphate, but noradrenergic inputs could only be expected to provide a spatially broad band activation of this second messenger system. VIP neurons might play a similar role but on a much finer spatial scale.

The need to process and distribute information about several different aspects of the stimulus simultaneously and to represent information at different spatial scales has imposed severe design constraints on the cortex. The laminar and surface organization of the cortex and its multiplicity of transmitter systems appear to represent efforts to solve these problems.

Further reading

Hendrickson AE (1985): Dots, stripes, and columns in monkey visual cortex. *Trend Neurosci* 9:406–410

Hubel DH, Wiesel TN (1977): Functional architecture of macacque monkey visual cortex. Ferrier Lecture *Proc R Soc Lond* (Biol) 198:1–59

Marr D (1982): *Vision*. San Francisco: Freeman

Parnavelas JG, MacDonald JK (1983): *The cereberal cortex.* In: *Chemical Neuroanatomy.* Emerson PC, ed. New York: Raven Press

Shaw C, Cynader M (1986): Laminar distribution of receptors in monkey (*Macaca fascucularis*) geniculastriate system. *J Comp Neurol,* 248:301–312

Visual Cortex, Extrastriate

David C. Van Essen

Extrastriate visual cortex comprises a mosaic of anatomically and physiologically distinct areas which occupy a broad belt of cortex outside the striate area (area 17, or V1). These areas receive their major visual input directly or indirectly from striate cortex and are responsible for intermediate and high levels of visual processing. Much research over the past 15 years has been directed at several general issues: (1) How many visual areas are there, and how can they be reliably identified? (2) How are these areas interconnected? (3) What types of visual information are processed within each area?

Number of areas

In every mammalian species that has been examined with modern anatomical and physiological techniques, many more visual areas have been identified than the three basic subdivisions proposed by Brodmann and other classical anatomists (i.e., areas 17, 18, and 19). Some of the additional areas lie within erstwhile areas 18 and 19, rendering these terms obsolete, while others are in the temporal, parietal, and frontal lobes.

In the macaque monkey, used as a representative here because it has been the most intensively studied, there are at least 15 cortical areas that are largely or exclusively visual in function. The location of these areas is shown in Figure 1 on a two-dimensional, unfolded map of the entire cerebral hemisphere. Each of these areas has been identified by criteria derived from one or more of the following experimental approaches: (1) mapping of the visual field representation across the surface of the cortex; (2) tracing of pathways to and from other cortical areas; (3) analysis of cortical myeloarchitecture; and (4) determination of the receptive field properties characteristic of cells in different areas. There is considerable variability from one hemisphere to the next in the size and position of each area, and precise delineation of boundaries is at present possible for only five visual areas (solid lines on figure; other boundaries indicated by dashed lines).

Eight of the identified visual areas in the macaque contain topographically organized representations of part or all of the contralateral visual hemifield. For some areas the representation is incomplete (e.g., only upper fields in the ventral posterior area, VP, and lower fields in V3), and in others (e.g., the middle temporal area, MT), the representation shows considerable local disorderliness. Beyond the areas illustrated in Figure 1 there is additional visually responsive cortex, and there are plausible candidates for several more visual, visuomotor, or polysensory areas. The total number of identifiable cortical areas closely related to vision in the macaque may eventually exceed 20.

Similar approaches have led to the identification of numerous visual areas in other species, including the owl monkey (a dozen or more areas), cat (up to 17 areas), and rat (at least 6 areas). In primates, a few areas, including V1, V2, and MT, are clearly present in all species studied, and there are several reasonable candidates for additional homologies. In contrast, unambiguous homologies between visual areas in primates and nonprimates have proved much more difficult to ascertain, except for V1 and V2.

Interconnections of visual areas

The application of modern anterograde and retrograde pathway-tracing techniques has led to the demonstration of a remarkably large number of corticocortical visual pathways as well as numerous connections with subcortical visual centers. Each visual area has multiple inputs and outputs. In the macaque, nearly all pathways conform to two organizational principles: they are organized in reciprocal fashion; and each reciprocal pair of connections is asymmetric in laminar organization, with the pathway having a pattern suggestive of feedforward inputs in one direction and feedback in the other. On this basis the identified visual areas in the macaque can be arranged in an anatomical hierarchy, in which each area occupies a well-defined level with respect to other areas (Fig. 2). In other species, reciprocity and asymmetric laminar patterns of corticocortical pathways are generally observed, suggesting that anatomically based hierarchical relationships may not be unique to the macaque.

Many corticocortical projections have been found to be organized in patchy fashion. The significance of this has been most clearly elucidated for area V2, which also has a characteristic internal pattern of stripes revealed by histochemical staining for cytochrome oxidase. The patchy projections from V1 to V2 and from V2 to V4 and MT are closely linked to the cytochrome oxidase stripes, suggesting that they provide a framework for modular organization akin to that which has been found for V1.

Functions of extrastriate areas

Lesion studies in primates and clinical observations in humans suggest that visual cortex in the temporal lobe is involved in high-level pattern recognition and form analysis (what an object is), whereas visual cortex in the parietal lobe is concerned with spatial relationships and visual attention (where objects of interest are). A major challenge for neurophysiology and neuroanatomy is to identify the areas and pathways contributing to these distinct functional streams and to determine the types of visual processing that occur at each level.

Single-unit recordings have demonstrated several types of functional specificity in extrastriate cortex. The most striking example is area MT, which contains a high percentage of cells selective for direction and speed of movement but relatively nonselective for form and color. The responses of cells in MT are modulated by moving patterns outside the classical

Figure 1. An unfolded two-dimensional map of cerebral cortex from the right hemisphere of a macaque monkey. The map is topologically equivalent to the intact cortical surface, except for one long discontinuity along the border between V1 and V2 and a shorter discontinuity in the frontal lobe. In addition to the 15 known visual areas, regions concerned with audition, somatic sensation, and motor control are indicated on the map. Abbreviations: AIT, anterior inferotemporal; LIP, lateral intraparietal; MST, medial superior temporal; MT, middle temporal; PIT, posterior inferotemporal; PO, parieto-occipital; VIP, ventral intraparietal; VP, ventral posterior.

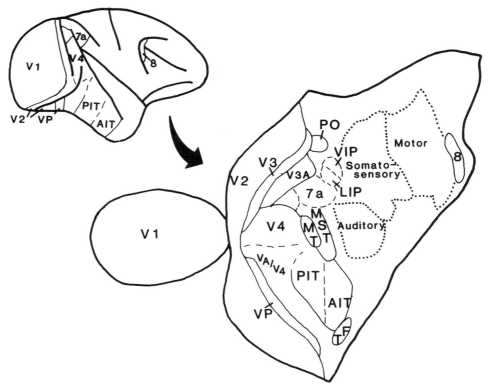

receptive field in a manner that may reflect the analysis of relative motion in the visual field. Also, some cells in macaque MT respond to complex moving patterns in a way indicative of a higher level of analysis than that occurring in V1. Additional evidence that MT is specifically involved in motion analysis comes from the behavioral effects of small chemically induced lesions, which perturb a monkey's ability to estimate the speed and direction of a moving spot.

In V4, roughly half the cells are color selective, and the responses of many of these are modulated by the illumination of regions surrounding the classical receptive field in a way that may contribute to the perceptual stability of colored objects under varied illumination conditions. Many cells in V4 are

orientation selective, and many cells in DL, the presumed homolog of V4 in the owl monkey, are highly selective for stimulus length and width. On these and other grounds, it is likely that V4 is heavily involved in the analysis of stimulus form as well as color. A surprising asymmetry in visual function has been found between V3, a lower field area which contains few color-selective cells but many direction-selective cells, and VP, an upper field area which contains many color-selective cells but few direction-selective cells.

V2 in the macaque contains many types of stimulus selectivity, but most of those reported (orientation, binocular disparity, color, and direction selectivity) are already encoded in V1. Most intriguing is the finding of cells in V2, but not V1, which respond to stimuli that evoke percepts of illusory contours in humans.

In inferotemporal cortex, a significant percentage of cells in certain subregions respond well to photographs or sketches of very complex stimuli such as faces or hands but poorly to much simpler stimuli. There remains a large gap between the relatively simple levels of form selectivity that have so far been demonstrated in lower areas (V2 and V4) and the much more advanced levels suggested by these results in inferotemporal cortex. Progress on these and related issues should markedly improve our understanding of the neural basis of complex perceptual processes.

Further reading

Ungerleider LG, Mishkin M (1982): Two cortical visual systems. In: *Analysis of Visual Behavior*, Ingle DJ, Goodale MA, Mansfield RJW, eds. Cambridge: MIT Press

Van Essen DC, Maunsell JHR (1983): Hierarchical organization and functional streams in the visual cortex. *Trends Neurosci* 6:370–375

Van Essen DC (1985): Functional organization of primate visual cortex. In: *Cerebral Cortex, Vol 3*, Peters A, Jones EG, eds. New York: Plenum Press, pp. 259–329.

Woolsey CN (1982): *Cortical Sensory Organization. Vol 2, Multiple Visual Areas*. Clifton NJ: Humana Press

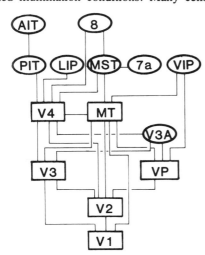

Figure 2. A proposed hierarchy of visual areas in the macaque. Unambiguously identified areas are enclosed by rectangles, whereas areas whose identification is tentative or uncertain are enclosed by ellipses. Lines interconnecting areas represent pathways which in most cases have been shown to be reciprocal (see Van Essen, 1985).

Visual Development, Infant

Richard Held

The question "What can infants see" has long intrigued laymen and scientists alike. In recent decades a surge of new results in vision research has deepened the importance of the question and begun to provide answers. Knowledge of the status of infants' vision, its development, and the underlying neuronal mechanisms is gained by noninvasive procedures, with the exceptions of anatomical studies of postmortem tissue. Otherwise, our knowledge has been based upon observations aided by instruments, psychophysical studies, and electrophysiology done with scalp electrodes. Inferences about neuronal mechanisms are often guided by physiological and anatomical knowledge obtained from animal studies, in particular, those performed on primates. In addition to its scientific interest, the study of normal and abnormal visual development is of clinical importance in interpreting the deleterious effects of early pathologies of significant incidence in infants, such as strabismus, anisometropia, high refractive errors, and congenital cataract.

Optics

Since the source of visual stimulation is light focused on the retinas, clarity of the ocular media is important. The light transmitting media in infants' eyes are normally clear at birth and remain so. Their refracting power, including accommodation of the lens, appears to be adequate for the relatively low levels of resolution that are achieved in infancy (discussed below). Infants' refraction differs from that of adults in showing a higher incidence of astigmatism (estimated range between 20% and 60%) on different axes, less myopia, and a lessened accommodative range during the very early months of life.

Eye motility

The retina forms part of the eye that can move. Eye movement has numerous consequences for vision. Primary among these is the ability to foveate targets in order to resolve fine detail. In the case of a moving field of objects, the eyes of an adult pursue the target to maintain foveation but, being limited in their amplitude of rotation, they periodically jerk back in the opposite direction by means of rapid saccades (optokinetic nystagmus). The pursuit mechanism appears to be adequate soon after birth for low velocity targets but fails for higher velocities, a state of affairs which improves with age and which may reflect the development of the fovea. Curiously enough, when one eye of an infant of less than three months of age is exposed to such targets, pursuit is adequate for motion in the temporal to nasal direction but grossly ineffective for the opposite direction of motion. Not until the fourth month on average is this asymmetry overcome. In the case of head movements, a vestibularly activated reflex rotates the eyes in the compensatory direction so as to hold fixation. This ability

appears to be present soon after birth. The combined orientations of the two eyes (vergence) determine the correspondence of the two retinal images and hence exert a limitation on stereopsis. Accurate vergence appears to develop over the first few months. Chronically inaccurate vergence of the two eyes is the condition called strabismus, some forms of which may cause amblyopia (a form of blindness) in infancy and lead to a permanent loss of binocularity.

Visual fields

Normal adults can detect stimuli at least 90 degrees off the optical axis of the eye on the temporal side and are limited on the nasal side only by the occluding effect of their noses. Newborn infants, however, have visual fields not extending more than 30 degrees from their optical axis. Moreover, they are more sensitive to stimuli on the temporal side. The extent of fields increases with age. It is not known whether these results reflect visual or attentional processes, or perhaps both.

Discrimination

The body of data on visual resolution obtained by the use of observational, psychophysical, and electrophysiological techniques is probably the most important source of information about the developing visual system of the infant. These techniques are designed to test for the detection and discrimination of stimuli. Perhaps most used is the preferential looking paradigm, which is based upon the original discovery that an infant will prefer to gaze in the direction of a region in its field of vision that is brighter, or has more edges, more motion, more solidity, more color, or more of some other property than other regions in the visual field. For example, an infant can be presented with a choice between a grating (typically one made up of alternating black and white bars of equal width) and a blank field of the same overall shape, average brightness, and color (Figure 1). When the bars are detectable, the infant will show gaze preference for them on repeated trials. The width of the bars can then be reduced in steps until the bars are no longer discriminable. The preference will have fallen to 50% (chance). The width of the bar at 75% preference is often taken as the threshold. Other properties of stimuli can be similarly varied in magnitude so as to obtain thresholds for other visual capacities.

Two types of visual capabilities can be distinguished on the basis of their developmental histories: those that are present at birth and appear to change little with age, and those that are either poor or absent at birth but improve or appear with increasing age. Among the former are brightness, color, motion, and temporal sensitivity; the latter include many forms of spatial resolution such as grating acuity, stereoacuity, and vernier acuity, several forms of binocular interaction including

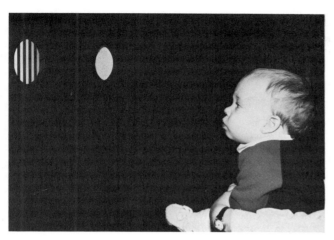

Figure 1. Preferential looking test with choice between grating and blank. Observer watches infant through peephole in screen.

rivalry, binocular summation, and susceptibility to amblyopia. The latter type yield more information relevant to the underlying neuronal mechanism since they show a course of development which can be related to that of neuronal mechanisms.

Grating acuity and contrast sensitivity

The most commonly used measure of resolution is the so-called minimum separable, that is, the smallest separation in the visual angle between two edges that can be detected. The reciprocal of this measurement is referred to as visual acuity. A set of equally spaced black and white bars that form a square-wave grating is a convenient stimulus for this purpose because its spatial periodicity can easily be specified in terms of the spatial frequency (repetitions per degree of visual angle) of its components. The acuity threshold is defined as the spatial frequency of the grating which is just detectable at high contrast. The related measure of contrast sensitivity is defined as the just detectable degree of contrast at specified spatial frequencies. Contrast sensitivity across the spatial frequency spectrum can in principle determine the visibility of any achromatic form which can be harmonically analyzed into its component frequencies and their phase relations.

Using variants of the forced-choice looking preference technique, results from several laboratories agree in showing that grating acuity in newborn infants has a spatial frequency of approximately one cycle per degree of visual angle (20/600 Snellen). It increases steadily in succeeding months such that acuity in cycles per degree is roughly equal to age in months over the first year. It reaches adult levels only after 7–10 years. Tests of preterm infants have shown that this development is closely related to conceptual age, rather than postnatal age, indicating that maturation is the important variable. The same techniques used to establish contrast sensitivity show an initial sensitivity of about one-thirtieth that of the adult level followed by a steady increase with age. The frequency of peak sensitivity increases from a fraction of a cycle to several cycles per degree over the first six months. These data are obtained by testing gratings with edges oriented either horizontally or vertically. Infants begin to show the lowered acuity for oblique relative to main axes gratings, observed in adults, by six months of age.

Amplitude measures of visually evoked potentials show initial levels of acuity roughly equal to those found by preferential looking, but the rate of increase is greater such that by six months infants show adult levels of acuity. The reasons for this discrepancy are not yet understood. On the other hand, latency measures of evoked potentials show a time course of change (reduction) similar to that of looking preference measures of acuity.

Stereopsis and binocularity

Several types of display have been used to test for stereopsis in infants. To distinguish discrimination of depth based upon stereopsis from that based upon other stimulus cues, random dot displays have been used. Alternatively, line stereograms can be used, provided that control displays demonstrate that the discrimination is, in fact, based upon stereopsis and not upon other cues to depth. Scalp potentials can be evoked by stereoptic displays. These methods yield similar results. They show an absence of stereopsis in the early months with an average onset age of four months and a range from two to six months. Additional studies show that the stereoacuity threshold rises to at least one minute of arc within a few weeks after onset of stereopsis. This abrupt rise contrasts radically with the development of grating acuity, which is present at birth and shows a relatively long slow rise with age. Since the neural signals from each of the two eyes do not converge functionally until they arrive in the visual cortex, development of that structure is suspected to underlie the onset of stereopsis and the rapid rise of stereoacuity.

Several other indices of binocularity have been developed. In the two-choice preference paradigm, stimuli which cause binocular rivalry in adult vision appear to be avoided by infants who have stereopsis. However, before the onset of stereopsis, very young infants show either no preferential response to fusible over rivalrous stimuli, or a clear preference for the rivalrous stimuli if superposition of its two views yield a figure that is more complex than the fused one. Nonselective combination of stimulus inputs to the two eyes seems to characterize vision prior to the onset of stereopsis. The transition to preference for the fused stimulus occurs at the same time as does the onset of stereopsis. Another finding which has been interpreted as an index of binocularity is the onset of binocular summation of the pupillary response. When light is available to only one eye, the pupil constricts to some constant level. When the same light is available to both eyes the pupil constricts a bit more, demonstrating binocular summation. Studies of infants show that such summation is weak in very young infants but increases to adult level by about four months of age, the same time as the onset of binocularity indices.

Vernier acuity

In adult observers the minimum separable acuity appears to have a lower limit of approximately a half minute determined by both the resolution of the optics of the eye and the grain of the receptor mosaic. However, considerably smaller spatial differences can be detected in certain configurations. These achievements constitute the so-called hyperacuities because they exceed the limitations on the minimum separable. For example, resolution for vernier offsets (slightly displaced segments of a straight edge) as small as a few seconds of visual angle can be detected by adult observers. The study of vernier acuity in infants has revealed that vernier acuity is initially less than grating acuity but, beginning in the fourth month, exceeds it. The crossing point appears to occur at the same time as the onset of stereopsis. If hyperacuity in infants is defined as resolution significantly better than grating acuity, then the capacity for hyperacuity has its onset during the fourth month. The vernier acuity results are in accord with those from the study of hyperacute stereopsis (high stereoacuity) which also has its onset at the same age. The agreement among onset times suggests concomitant developments in the visual cortex.

Clinical relevance

During the 1960s and 1970s physiological and anatomical studies of the visual cortex in animals yielded unusually clear demonstrations of the interacting roles of maturation and exposure to the visual environment in determining the development of the visual system. Occlusion of one eye during a sensitive period early in life was shown to alter radically the central connections within cortex as well as to reduce visual function. Similar consequences were shown to follow from early strabismus. These results are relevant to analogous human pathologies such as early occlusive cataract and congenital strabismus. What is the sensitive period during which the infant may lose visual function under the conditions that are known to alter the visual nervous system? Use of new measurements of acuity has begun to reveal the onset of at least one sensitive period, i.e., the development of amblyopia resulting from esotropia (cross-eyedness in which one eye turns inward). Its earliest appearance occurs in the third or fourth month, roughly the same age as the development of binocularity. Acuity measurements have also revealed the effects of monocular occlusion therapy used for correcting the amblyopia. When the nonamblyopic eye is chronically patched, the amblyopic eye often shows an improved acuity but at the cost of a reduction of acuity in the patched eye. This reciprocity is characteristic of the effects of occlusion during the sensitive period which appears to extend throughout the early years of childhood.

In addition to this clinical relevance, measuring procedures are finding direct application in two forms. First, these new tests can assess the status of the vision of infants suspected to be at risk for early pathology. Second, they can assess the visual consequences of therapy and be used to titrate the amounts of chronic treatments such as occlusion therapy.

Neuronal mechanisms

Many changes in relevant neuronal paths and nuclei occur during the infant's growth. The most obvious are changes in the anatomy of the retina, particularly in the region of the fovea, myelination of neurons in the optic nerve and elsewhere, and changes in cortex. Anatomical change in the fovea may increase the packing density of receptors and hence increase resolution. Changes in cortex, such as segregation of the ocular dominance columns, may account for the onset of binocularity. The search for the neuronal correlates of visual development continues.

Further reading

Aslin RN, Alberts JR, Petersen MR, eds (1981): *Development of Perception: Psychobiological Perspectives. Vol 2: The Visual System.* In: *Behavioral Biology*, JL McGaugh, JC Fentress, and JP Hegmann, series eds. New York: Academic Press

Atkinson J (1984): Human visual development over the first 6 months of life: A review and a hypothesis. *Human Neurobiol* 3:61–74

Behav Brain Res (1983): Special issue on development of visual functions in infants and children 10:1

Preparation of this review was supported in part by a grant from the National Institutes of Health (No. 2 RO1-EY 01191).

Visual Field

Ernst Pöppel

The visual field refers to the number of degrees of visual angle during stable fixation of the eyes. Monocular measurement of the visual field by perimetry, shows that the left and the right half of the visual field are not the same size. The temporal visual field, extending from the vertical meridian toward the periphery, is considerably larger than the nasal visual field. Measurements along the horizontal meridian show that targets even beyond 90° eccentricity can be detected on the temporal side; the limit of light detection is 50–60° on the nasal side. The upper and lower halves of the visual field appear to be equal, with the limits at approximately 50–60° eccentricity, although there are large individual differences. If the visual fields of the two eyes are superimposed as in normal vision, the binocular visual field covers more than 180° along the horizontal meridian. The most eccentric part of the temporal visual field that lies beyond the border of the nasal visual field of the other eye is called monocular crescent. Thus, binocular vision is provided only up to the border of the nasal visual field; the far periphery on the left and right side is seen monocularly.

Visual field measurements are usually done using a white test target of high contrast that is moved from the periphery toward the center of the visual field. If instead light-difference threshold is measured at various positions of the visual field of one eye using a stationary target (static perimetry) in addition to visual field extent, local sensitivity can be determined. Under photopic adaptation conditions, the fovea centralis has the highest sensitivity. The perifoveal region is characterized by a decreasing sensitivity beginning at the fovea and ending approximately at 10° eccentricity. Beyond this there is a plateau of constant sensitivity that extends up to approximately 35° eccentricity on the temporal side and up to 20° eccentricity on the nasal side. Beyond this plateau, sensitivity again decreases until the end of the visual field. The blind spot lies within the plateau region on the temporal side, approximately between 14° and 18° eccentricity along the horizontal meridian (Fig. 1). Under scotopic adaptation, the fovea and perifoveal region are less sensitive than the more peripheral regions of the retina because of the shift from cone-dominated to rod-dominated vision. If a colored target instead of a white target is used for visual field measurement, subjects are able to detect the target as it is moved from the periphery toward the center of the visual field at greater eccentricities than they can identify its color.

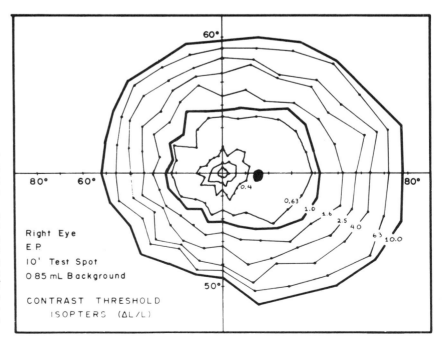

Figure 1. Light-difference threshold ($\Delta L/L$) isopters for the right eye of E.P., determined with a 10-min arc target. The target was presented for 200 msec on a 0.85 millilambert background. The visual field is represented in polar coordinates with the fovea at the origin. Horizontal and vertical meridians are marked at 10°; the contrast for the isopters is shown in the right lower quadrant. The contrast for the foveal vision under these conditions (for the right eye of E.P.) is 0.1. The isopters are based on measurements along 12 meridians. The measurements along each meridian were obtained in steps of 2° visual angle from the fovea to the limits of the visual field. Note the plateau of constant light—difference threshold surrounding the foveal and perifoveal region with its pronounced extension into the temporal visual field (nasal retina).

Although sensitivity varies throughout the visual field, apparent brightness remains constant under photopic adaptation; it does not get darker toward the periphery of the visual field. Constancy of brightness throughout the visual field can be demonstrated by using a visual target of constant contrast that is above threshold for all eccentricities tested; it is then scaled with respect to its apparent brightness by the technique of magnitude estimation. Apparent brightness is directly related to the physical energy of the visual stimulus and not to local sensitivity of the retina. (Note that this observation disproves Fechner's law as far as accounting for brightness perception throughout the visual field.) Under scotopic adaptation, constancy of brightness throughout the visual field is observed only for the periphery; in order for foveal and perifoveal targets to appear equally bright they must have a higher contrast. For constancy of brightness one has to assume a neuronal mechanism that compensates for the changing sensitivity of the retina as a function of eccentricity. It is still unclear where and how such a mechanism might work although it has been suggested that it is already implemented at the retinal level.

If the two eyes are properly aligned while fixating an object, each position in binocular visual space is represented at corresponding retinal points. In case of a misalignment, i.e., if the two visual axes are uncorrelated, a point in space is represented at noncorresponding retinal points. Such a deviation of the visual axes may result in the experience of double images, because the visual fields of the two eyes no longer coincide. Proper alignment of the eyes is necessary for stereoscopic vision; if not corrected in early childhood misalignment may result in a loss of stereoscopic vision and the reduction of sensitivity in one eye.

How is the visual field represented in the brain (Fig. 2)? The first observation on visual field representation may already go back to Descartes who discovered that left and right and top and bottom of an object are reversed on the retina. Thus, the temporal visual field of each eye is represented on the nasal half of the retina, and the nasal visual field on the temporal retina. If one fixates an object and draws a vertical line through the fixation point, everything that is to the left of this line is represented on the nasal half of the retina of the left eye and on the temporal half of the retina of the right eye. Everything to the right of this line is represented on the nasal retina of the right eye and on the temporal retina of the left eye.

The output of retinal information processing is collected in approximately 1 million ganglion cells whose axons form the optic nerve. The optic nerve leaves the eye at the optic disk that corresponds perceptually to the blind spot in the visual field. The optic nerve is split into halves at the optic chiasm. Those axons that carry information from the nasal retina cross over to the other side of the brain and those axons coming from the temporal retina stay on the same side. The fiber bundle beyond the optic chiasm, the optic tract, contains the information that comes from the nasal retina of one eye and the temporal retina of the other.

Most of the fibers coming from the retina project to the lateral geniculate nucleus (LGN), a subcortical brain structure with six layers each innervated by either the right or the left eye. Neurons in adjacent positions in the different layers are innervated by retinal fibers that represent corresponding retinal points of the two eyes. The representation of the retina in the LGN is retinotopic, i.e., the spatial structure of an object in visual space is preserved through the retina to the LGN, although within the optic nerve and the optic tract such retinotopy appears to be absent.

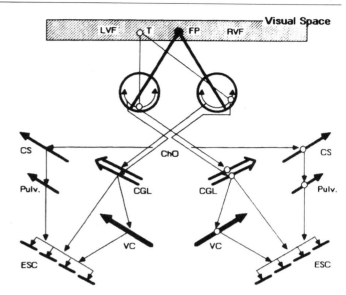

Figure 2. Schematic representation of major projections of visual space into the brain. FP, fixation point; LVF, RVF, left, right visual field; T, target presented in visual space; ChO, optic chiasm; CGL, corpus geniculatum laterale; VC, visual cortex; CS, superior colliculus; Pulv., pulvinar system; ESC, extrastriate cortex. Arrows indicate topological (retinotopic) representations; interhemispheric and efferent connections have been omitted.

The LGN projects to the striate cortex via the optic radiation, and the visual field representation in the striate cortex (also called visual cortex, area 17, occipital lobe, or V 1) retains its retinotopy. At the striate cortex, the separate representations of the visual field in the different layers of the LGN are fused into one visual field representation by way of binocular innervation of cortical neurons. The specific retinotopic representation of the visual field in humans has been mapped with the help of brain-injured patients who have suffered total or partial lesions of the striate cortex. The total loss of striate cortex within one hemisphere results in a complete homonymous hemianopia. A patient with such a condition has no vision in the temporal visual field of one eye and in the nasal visual field of the other. Often, such patients show a foveal sparing, which suggests that the fovea of each eye is represented in both hemispheres.

Although the representation of the visual field at the striate cortex is retinotopic, the cortex does not devote equal neuronal space to equal visual space. The foveal and perifoveal region get much greater emphasis than the periphery, and this fact is expressed by way of the so-called magnification factor. More neuronal machinery is provided for the foveal and perifoveal region of the retina: ganglion cells in the retina are much more densely packed in that region that processes information at and closely to the visual axis, and each ganglion cell innervates via the LGN a roughly equal area of striate cortex.

The striate cortex is surrounded by secondary areas that are also concerned with visual information processing. These extrastriate areas appear to be specialized for the analysis of particular categories of visual information like depth, movement, or color. There is evidence from anatomical and physiological studies on nonhuman primates also supported by neuropsychological results obtained with brain-injured patients that a particular extrastriate region of extrastriate cortex (V 4) is concerned with color vision.

The visual field is also mapped onto the superior colliculus. With an injury in the geniculostriatal pathway, this retinal projection usually remains intact. This is why it has been suggested that blindsight may be mediated by the retinocollicular pathway, although other explanations are possible. The collicular representation of the visual field is probably also essential for the programming of saccadic eye movements. It is conceivable that a visual stimulus from the periphery of the visual field elicits directly a proper saccade on the basis of the collicular representation alone without involving the cortical representation. Thus, the superior colliculus has been considered an important link between the sensory representation of the visual field and the oculomotor system.

Further reading

Aulhorn E, Harms H (1972): Visual perimetry. In: *Handbook of Sensory Physiology 7/4* Jameson D, Hurvich LM, eds. Berlin: Springer-Verlag

Hubel DH, Wiesel TN (1977): Functional architecture of macaque visual cortex. *Proc R Soc Lond* B 198:1–59

Polyak S (1957): *The Vertebrate Visual System*. Chicago: University of Chicago Press

Pöppel E, Held R, Dowling JE (1977): Neuronal mechanisms in visual perception. *Neurosci Res Prog Bull* 15:315–553

Pöppel E, Harvey LD Jr (1973): Light-difference threshold and subjective brightness in the periphery of the visual field. *Psychol Forschung* 36:145–161

Teuber H-L, Battersby WS, Bender MB (1960): *Visual Field Defects after Penetrating Missile Wounds of the Brain*. Cambridge: Harvard University Press

Visual Learning, Pattern and Form Perception: Central Mechanisms

Howard C. Hughes and James M. Sprague

It seems clear that our progress in understanding the neural subsystems underlying form and pattern vision will depend to a large extent on precise formulations of the manner in which forms and patterns are perceived in the first place. Over the last 20 years, two different modes of image processing have received the most attention. The first approach is known as hierarchical feature processing. According to this view, the visual system analyzes images by detecting the presence of local features (e.g., edges, line segments, and corners). Recognition then depends on the assimilation of these features into higher order groups that represent the boundaries of objects present in the scene. Interpretations of stimulus-induced activity of cortical cells in terms of feature detectors is consistent with this view, although it is generally recognized that individual cortical cells do not behave as true feature detectors (since, for example, there is a trade-off between orientation and contrast such that an optimally oriented bar of low contrast can produce the same response as a higher contrast bar in a different orientation). In any case, the notion of hierarchical feature detection logically leads to the idea that complicated percepts are encoded by individual neurons located at a "high level" in the visual system. Despite some evidence for such neurons in the inferotemporal cortex of monkeys, this approach is generally regarded as too cumbersome to provide the neural substrate of pattern and form vision in general, although this might be the way in which images of particular ecological relevance to an animal might be encoded.

The major alternative to feature detection is the suggestion that the visual system performs some type of spectral analysis (extracts spatial frequency components) of patterns. There is a great deal of psychophysical evidence consistent with this view, and the behavior of individual cortical cells can be interpreted as an orientation-specific, spatiotemporal band pass filter. The outputs of these filters presumably must be recombined at some later stage, but how this may be accomplished remains unclear. In addition, the issue of whether cortical neurons are best characterized as either line or edge detectors or spatial frequency filters remains controversial.

Historical background

Scientific study of the perceptual contributions of different parts of the central visual pathways of mammals has been ongoing for nearly a century. Throughout most of this period, the visual cortex has been taken as the sine qua non of form and pattern perception. According to this view, subcortical visual structures are relegated to performing more or less simple visual reflexes, such as the pupillary reflex, optokinetic nystagmus, and the visual orienting reflex involving head and eye movements. In visual perception, subcortical structures were thought to be limited to discrimination of gross differences in luminous flux. It was generally held that with the elaboration of the neocortex characteristic of mammals, the cortex had come to dominate functions performed by subcortical structures in submammalian forms. Recent studies in mammals, however, have indicated a major role of the superior colliculus in selective attention, in orientation, in the generation of saccadic eye movements, and, because of these functions, in pattern discrimination.

Stages of cortical processing

Until the mid-1960s, it was believed that the projections from the dorsal lateral geniculate nucleus (LGNd) provided the only pathway through which visual information could gain access to the cortex. Because the anatomical evidence indicated that in the primate, the cortical projections of the LGNd were confined to the striate cortex (Brodmann's area 17), this cortex, with its fine-grained retinotopic representation of the visual world, was viewed as the first stage in the cortical processing of visual information. As such, the striate cortex was considered the primary visual cortex. Visual areas beyond area 17 (e.g., areas 18 and 19) were considered association areas, meaning that they received their sole visual input from area 17, operating on this input to produce higher order visual function.

The assumption that the striate cortex represented the first stage in the serial processing of visual information in the cortex justified the use of large lesions in behavioral work, for under this assumption, incidental damage to the extrastriate visual areas was unimportant as long as the striate cortex was completely removed and the LGNd was completely atrophied. The concept of a serial hierarchy of cortical processes also related to the structuralist doctrine in sensory psychology. This doctrine held that complex percepts were constructed from lower order elementary sensations in striate cortex. This process of constructing percepts could produce emergent properties that were not present in the elementary sensations from which they arose, and was thought to occur in the extrastriate association areas.

The related ideas of structuralism and a serial hierarchy of cortical areas beginning with the primary area and proceeding through the association areas fit nicely with empirical findings indicating that damage to the visual cortex in primates produced profound blindness. These effects were attributed to striate damage, and the most concise statement of the visual capacities was that animals deprived of striate cortex could only detect differences in luminous flux; the capacity to discriminate patterns that differed in spatial distribution of luminous flux was thought to be absent. In humans, the consequences of striate damage were regarded as more severe, producing a homonomous hemianopia with complete damage in one hemisphere, and a circumscribed region of blindness (a scotoma) with subtotal damage. The visual coordinates of the scotoma corresponded to the portion of the visuotopic map that suffers the damage. The degree of blindness was thought to be as profound as that which follows a retinal lesion.

Parallel thalamocortical pathways

The idea that complete removal of all visually responsive neocortex results in pattern and form blindness is not seriously questioned, and the characterization of visually decorticate subjects as simple detectors of luminous flux is probably accurate. As to the primacy of area 17, however, it is now well established that the model outlined here is incorrect. Opposing evidence comes from a large number of behavioral studies that show that the consequences of damage restricted to area 17 are much less severe than those that follow larger lesions. In addition, it is also clear that damage to the extrastriate cortex leads to important visual disturbances even when the striate cortex is intact. This reevaluation of the behavioral effects of damage to the visual cortex was spurred by anatomical findings that have revolutionized our understanding of the cortical organization of sensory systems. The extrastriate cortex receives a subcortical afferent supply independent of the geniculostriate system. This pathway, which exists in all species examined thus far, includes the well-known retinal projection to the superior colliculus, a newly discovered ascending projection from the colliculus to the pulvinar complex of the thalamus, and from there to the extrastriate cortex. The existence of this pathway led workers to attempt lesions limited to the striate cortex, and thus the extensive visual abilities of destriate animals came to be appreciated. Moreover, with the importance of the extrastriate cortex established behaviorally, electrophysiologists began to study the extrastriate areas in more detail, which led to the discovery of multiple, retinotopic representations within the visual association areas. The anatomical interconnections between these different areas are complex and difficult to characterize succinctly. One important point should be made clear, however: the geniculocortical and colliculopulvinar cortical pathways are not strictly independent. Both corticofugal and corticopetal cross-talk occurs. For example, the superior colliculus projects to LGNd as well as to pulvinar. In addition, the pulvinar projects to area 17 while the lateral geniculate projects to the extrastriate as well as the striate cortex. In terms of corticofugal projections, both striate and extrastriate cortex project subcortically to the superior colliculus, pulvinar, and LGNd. Thus, damage to any component of the central visual system may produce changes in the operation of remaining structures in addition to system changes that result from the specific structure damaged. This presents problems in interpreting the consequences of brain damage and in localization of functions, but important facts can nonetheless be established. First, the absence of a deficit can, under certain circumstances, be important and informative, provided that the behavioral tests have demonstrable sensitivity. In this context, psychophysical testing can be useful. Second, strong inferences can be gained if damage to one component produces a deficit on one task and not on another, while damage to a different component produces the inverse. This is called a double dissociation of results and can be used to make strong functional inferences from lesion experiments.

Vision in the absence of striate cortex

The modern view of the functional organization of the striate cortex grew primarily from the famous collaboration between David Hubel and Torsten Wiesel. Their work made it clear that the striate cortex performs a piecemeal analysis of the visual scene. It is possible to view the striate cortex as performing a sorting operation in which each local region of visual space is analyzed in terms of several lower level stimulus dimensions, and the results of this processing are transmitted to other portions of the visual system. It is clear that spatial interactions of adjacent regions within the striate cortex are limited. Thus, if form and pattern vision depend on appreciation of spatial structure distributed over large areas of the retina, it is unlikely that form recognition occurs in area 17. It seems more likely that the mechanisms of form perception are in areas where precise retinotopic organization has given way to a broader, more global representation of visual space, such as in the temporal or parietal areas. It clearly remains possible that these extrastriate areas depend on area 17 for their input. The degree of this dependence varies across species. The consequences of striate damage seem most severe in primates, especially humans.

In cats, removal of areas 17 and 18, with complete loss of the *x-cell* pathway, has remarkably little impact on visually guided behavior. Visual perimetry in destriate cats indicates that the visual fields are full and intact: there is no evidence of homonomous hemianopia following unilateral lesions, and no indications of scotoma following subtotal lesions. In addition, the basic mechanisms of form and pattern perception clearly do not depend on areas 17 and 18, as there is no loss of preoperatively learned discriminations.

Psychophysical data indicate that destriate cats show losses in visual acuity that are modest for grating acuity but more severe for vernier acuity; these functions require high resolution and probably depend on the x-cell pathway. The dissociation between acuity and pattern and form perception is interesting, as it implies that acuity is not particularly important unless the discrimination requires good resolution (and many do not). This dissociation may relate to a growing appreciation of the importance of low-resolution processes in pattern and form vision which probably relate chiefly to function of the *y-cell* pathway. As the general shapes of objects and patterns are frequently specified by their low spatial frequency content, the suggestion has been made that low-resolution processes may provide an important input for the mechanisms of pattern and form vision. Indeed, under certain circumstances, low-frequency information seems to dominate cues represented by higher spatial frequencies. The so-called global precedence effect may represent one manifestation of this idea. In any case, the relationship between good pattern and form vision and a sensitivity to low spatial frequencies, where the y cells tend to be especially sensitive, finds additional support in the finding that destriate cats demonstrate reduced contrast sensitivity to high- but not low-frequency gratings. Finally, it should be mentioned that striate removal produces impairments in depth perception, and probably deficient stereoscopic vision.

What structures support pattern and form vision in the absence of area 17? If removal of areas 17 and 18 has so little impact on a cat's visually guided behavior, what neural structures are important? As we have indicated, complete ablation of all visual areas within the cortex does indeed produce profound form and pattern blindness and, if done unilaterally, homonomous hemianopia. In addition, extrastriate visual areas receive afferent pathways that are independent of the connection with area 17 and that arise from the lateral geniculate and colliculorecipient division of the pulvinar. Cats with lesions of the extrastriate cortex (sparing 17 and 18) show prolonged learning on the same patterns and form discriminations that are unaffected by striate damage. Thus, the suggestion has been made that, in cats, the neural mechanisms that subserve pattern and form vision depend more on the extrastriate than the striate cortex. These same extrastriate cortical areas are responsible for interhemispheric transfer of form discriminations. Moreover, visual acuity in these extrastriate animals is not impaired. Thus, a double dissociation between the striate and extrastriate cortex has been established: striate lesions produce an acuity deficit while leaving form and pattern vision largely unaffected and the converse applies to extensive extrastriate damage.

Destriate vision in primates and humans

The situation in primates differs somewhat from that described for cats. In rhesus monkeys, removal of the striate cortex produces hemianopia, and transient scotomas in more circumscribed lesions. Preoperatively learned pattern and form discriminations are lost postoperatively, but can be relearned with extensive practice. These visual abilities are appropriately considered residual, i.e., they are normally mediated by striate cortex, but can be relearned without it. Following recovery, destriate monkeys seem to possess a great deal of visual capacity: they do not bump into objects and seem to get along pretty well. They can learn pure form discriminations (i.e., discriminations between stimuli that are equated in their amount of contour, total luminous flux, and size). They are amblyopic, however, as demonstrated by reduced contrast sensitivity for all spatial frequencies.

The effects of striate removal in macaques are clearly more severe than those found in cats. Although the reasons for the differences are not clear, a reasonable hypothesis can be suggested. Cats possess extensive geniculate input to the extrastriate cortex, so that the y-cell pathway reaches most of the multiple visual cortical areas. On the other hand, both the y-cell and the x-cell pathways in monkeys terminate solely in the striate cortex. This primate characteristic of increasing importance of the striate cortex is even more pronounced in humans, where striate damage has catastrophic effects for the individual. Extensive unilateral damage to the striate cortex in humans produces a contralateral homonomous hemianopia, and subtotal damage produces a dense scotoma. Thus, when visual stimuli are presented within a hemianopic field, affected individuals do not report visual sensations. These effects have been known for 70 years and probably contributed to the confusion that characterized early animal studies. Interestingly, more recent animal experiments led investigators to reevaluate the possibility of residual visual functions in destriate humans us-

ing forced alternative techniques similar to those used in animal studies. In this procedure, subjects know that a stimulus will be presented and have to choose (or guess) which of two alternative stimuli was presented. In tests of visual localization, they must guess the location of the stimulus, rather than report whether or not they saw it. The general finding that has emerged from these studies is that although subjects cannot report on or describe stimuli presented in their blind fields, they can frequently guess correctly at rates far above those expected on the basis of chance alone. Since this performance apparently occurs in the absence of awareness, the phenomenon has been called *blindsight*. It has recently been suggested that the blindsight phenomenon might be an artifact of stray light or severely amblyopic vision supported by residual striate tissue. Thus, the issue of residual vision in destriate humans remains unresolved, at least in the minds of some workers. Ultimate resolution of this conflict of interpretation will have to await additional testing in these patients as well as histological verification of their lesions. The issue has obvious clinical importance and could also help further our understanding of the role of the retinocollicular-pulvinar-extrastriate system in human vision.

Further reading

Cats

Berkley MA, Sprague JM (1979): Striate cortex and visual acuity functions in the cat. *J Comp Neurol* 187:679–702

Sherman SM (1986): Functional organization of the w-, x-, and y-cell pathways in the cat: A review and hypothesis. In: *Progress in Psychobiology and Physiological Psychology*, vol 11, Sprague JM, Epstein AN, eds. New York: Academic Press

Sprague JM, Hughes HC, Berlucchi G (1981): Cortical Mechanisms in Pattern and Form Perception. In: *Brain Mechanisms and Perceptual Awareness*, Pompeiano O, Ajmone Marsan C, eds. New York: Raven Press

Monkeys

Pasik P, Pasik T (1982): Visual functions in monkeys after total removal of the visual cerebral cortex. In: *Contributions to Sensory Physiology*, Neff WD, ed. New York: Academic Press

Humans

Campion L, Latto R, Smith M (1983): Is blindsight an effect of scattered light, spared cortex, and near threshold vision? *Behav Brain Sci* 6:423–486

Weiskrantz L (1980): Varieties of residual experience. *Q J Exp Psychol* 32:365–386

Visual Motion Perception

Shimon Ullman

The use of visual motion

Visual motion provides useful information about the surrounding environment, and this information is extracted and used by biological visual systems in a variety of tasks. Sophisticated mechanisms for extracting and utilizing visual motion are found even in simple animals. For example, the frog has efficient "bug detection" mechanisms that respond selectively to small dark objects moving in its visual field. The ordinary housefly can track moving objects and can discover the relative motion between a target and its background when the two are identical in texture and therefore indistinguishable in the absence of relative motion. Visual motion is also used in the guidance of locomotion and the control of body motion. Another remarkable use of visual motion is the interpretation of structure from motion, which is the recovery of three-dimensional shape using motion information alone. This capacity has been demonstrated in the classical studies of H. Wallach and D.N. O'Connell, in which an unfamiliar object was rotated behind a translucent screen and its shadow projection observed from the other side of the screen. The viewers were able to give a correct description of the hidden object's three-dimensional structure and motion in space, even when each static view was unrecognizable and contained no three-dimensional information.

In view of the central role of motion perception, it is not surprising that the analysis of visual motion is wired into the system from the earliest processing stages. In some species, including the pigeon and the rabbit, rudimentary motion analysis is performed as early as the retinal level. At the level of the primary visual cortex in the cat and monkey many of the neurons are already involved in the analysis of motion: they respond well to stimuli moving in one direction, but little or not at all to motion in the opposite direction.

There are two main areas of problems in motion perception: the measurement of motion and the interpretation of visual motion. Only the first of these will be discussed here. For a discussion of the interpretation problem (e.g., the use of motion information to recover the three-dimensional structure of objects) see Ullman (1979).

Measuring visual motion

The primary problem in motion perception is that motion in the image is not given directly, but must be computed from more elementary measurements. Psychophysical evidence in recent years has advanced the view that two different mechanisms are involved in motion detection and measurement: short range and long range. The short-range mechanism measures continuous motion, or motion presented discretely with spatial displacements of up to about 15 min of arc (in the center of the visual field) and temporal intervals of less than about 60–100 msec. The long-range mechanism can process larger displacements and temporal intervals. Under the appropriate spatial and temporal presentation parameters, it can fill in the gaps in a discrete presentation of stimuli even when the stimuli are separated by up to several degrees of visual angle, and by long temporal intervals (400 msec and more). The resulting motion, termed apparent or beta motion can be perceptually indistinguishable from continuous motion.

The distinction between the two systems is more fundamental than their difference in range. The short-range process operates more directly on changes in the local light intensity distribution. The long-range process proceeds by first identifying image features such as line termination, corners, blobs, and regions, and then matching these features over time.

Short-range process of motion measurement

At least two intensity-based schemes have been advanced as models for motion measurement in biological systems. The first scheme compares the outputs of two detectors of light increments at two adjacent positions. The output at position p_1 and time t is compared with that of position p_2 at time $t - \delta t$ (low-pass temporal filtering can be employed instead of the temporal delay). Several variations of this scheme have been proposed. The first is obtained by multiplying the two values, i.e., $D(p_1, t) \cdot D(p_2, t - \delta t)$, where D denotes the output of the subunits. An alternative is the "and-not" scheme proposed by H. Barlow and R.W. Levick for directionally selective neurons in the rabbit's retina. In this scheme motion from p_2 to p_1 will be vetoed by the delayed inhibition from p_2, whereas motion from p_1 to p_2 will produce a positive response.

A different scheme for the detection and measurement of motion has been proposed as a model for motion analysis by cortical simple cells. This scheme is based on the combined measurement of intensity gradients and temporal changes. It uses the ratio between the temporal and spatial rates of change in the image to infer image velocities. This scheme is especially useful near objects' edges where relatively steep intensity gradients are induced.

At present, there is insufficient evidence to determine whether either of these schemes is actually employed by primate visual cortex.

Integration of motion measurements

Either one of these schemes can be used to determine motion of edge segments. An additional problem arises, however, since the motion of edges and contours cannot be determined on the basis of purely local measurements. The reason for this is the so-called aperture problem: if the motion is to be detected by a unit that is small compared to the overall length of the contour, the only information that can be extracted is the motion component perpendicular to the local orientation of the element. Motion along the element would be invisible. To determine the motion completely, a second stage that combines local measurements, either in local neighborhoods, or along the contour, is required. An integration scheme that solves this problem has been proposed recently by E. Hildreth. The scheme determines the velocity field from the initial measurements by minimizing the variation in the velocity field along image contours.

Long-range correspondence

The apparent motion phenomenon illustrates the visual system's capacity to establish visual motion by matching features over considerable spatial distances and temporal intervals. In perceiving continuous motion between successively presented elements, the visual system is faced with the difficult problem of establishing a correspondence between the elements of the two presentations. That is, for each element in the first frame, its counterpart in the subsequent frame must be located. The rules governing the correspondence process in human vision have been investigated extensively, but they are still only partially understood.

Neurophysiology of motion measurement

In primates, electrophysiological studies have identified directionally selective cells in a variety of visual areas. In addition, an area termed MT has been identified in the macaque monkey that seems to be specialized in the analysis of motion. Directionally selective units in V1 area appear to be involved primarily with short-range analysis. Little is known at present about the long-range process at the neurophysiological level. One obvious question is just where in the visual system apparent motion phenomena can be observed in the response of single units. Initial results suggest that units in MT may play a role in the perception of long-range apparent motion. MT seems also to be implicated in the integration of visual motion. J.A. Movshon has reported the existence of MT neurons that respond to the true two-dimensional direction of motion of visual patterns, unlike neurons in V1 that respond only to the movement component along the cell's preferred direction. It seems, in conclusion, that reasonable directions for further investigation at the neurophysiological level include the mechanisms underlying directional selectivity, the processes that integrate the initial local motion measurements, and the initial detection of long-range motion.

Further reading

Grusser O-J, Grusser-Cornehls U (1973): Neuronal mechanisms of visual movement perception and some psychophysical and behavioral correlation. In: *Handbook of Sensory Physiology*, Vol 7/3A:333–429, Jung R, ed. Berlin: Springer-Verlag

Hildreth EC (1983): *The Measurement of Visual Motion*. Cambridge: MIT Press

Kolers PA (1972): *Aspects of Motion Perception*. New York: Pergamon Press

Ullman S (1979): *The Interpretation of Visual Motion*. Cambridge: MIT Press

Visual Perception

Jeremy M. Wolfe

The stimulus for vision

The physical stimulus for vision is light, the band of electromagnetic radiation with wavelengths between 400 and 700 nm. The visual system can respond to a very large range of stimulus intensities. A single photon can have a measurable effect. The most intense light that can be viewed without damage to the eyes is 10^{13} times more intense than the dimmest visible light. Perceived brightness of a spot of light is not a linear function of its physical intensity. Brightness is roughly proportional to the cube root of intensity. To double the apparent brightness, intensity must be increased about tenfold. Of the 360 degrees around the head, a human's visual field covers more than 180 degrees horizontally and about 100 degrees vertically. Certain animals such as rabbits and frogs can see a full 360 degrees, but with a loss of the overlap between the visual fields of the two eyes.

Basic steps in visual perception

There are three major steps between a stimulus in the physical world and its visual perception:

1. An image of that stimulus is formed on the retina, the neural tissue at the back of the eye, and converted to electrochemical signals that can be processed by the nervous system.
2. Basic features such as color, size, and motion are extracted from that input.
3. Inferences are made about the nature of the real-world stimulus based on the processed input and the observer's knowledge about the visual world.

From light to visual system input

The optics place on the retina a two-dimensional pattern of light and dark. It is in continuous motion due to eye movements. Because of optical defects, the image is imperfectly focused and subject to chromatic aberration. This flat, moving, degraded image is the input to the visual system. Nevertheless, we see a three-dimensional, stable, sharp visual world filled with identifiable objects doing recognizable things. The task of the visual system is to make visual perception out of visual input.

As a first step, light is converted to electrochemical signals by the bleaching of pigment in two types of photoreceptors. Each type mediates different aspects of vision. The cones work in daylight (photopic), support color vision, and are most concentrated in the fovea (the part of the retina that is stimulated by an object in the direct line of sight). The rods work in dim illumination (scotopic), do not support color vision, and are absent in the central fovea. Visual acuity, the ability to resolve small details, is best in the fovea and gets rapidly worse as stimuli are moved away from the point of fixation. Since there are relatively few rods in the foveal region, visual acuity is markedly reduced under scotopic lighting conditions.

Extraction of basic visual features

The extraction of information from the retinal image takes place in several stages. The processing of size and color information begins in the retina itself. Lateral inhibitory interactions give rise to cells that respond optimally to light or dark spots of different size. The output of these cells can be used to locate the position of edges in the image. Illusions such as Mach bands and the Hermann grid are by-products of the processing of size and contour.

Similar interactions between three different types of cones give rise to cells differentially sensitive to the color of a stimulus. The three cone types are most sensitive to short (bluish), medium (greenish), and long (reddish) wavelengths of light. Inhibition between these types gives rise to three opponent mechanisms. One specifies where the stimulus lies on a continuum from red to green. Another does the same for the blue-yellow continuum, and the third for the black-white. Looking at one color can change the appearance of others. Thus, looking at a red light bleaches the long wavelength cones more than the others. This reduces sensitivity to red and alters the red-green opponent mechanism in such a way that previously white stimuli will look slightly green.

Further on the visual pathway, probably in visual cortex, the orientation of contours and their direction of motion are found. Taking orientation as an example, the orientation of a line is found by filtering the input through broadly tuned orientation channels. A channel is a psychophysical term referring to a mechanism that is sensitive to some stimuli but not others. An orientation channel tuned for vertical orientations would respond best to a vertical contour, less well to lines tilted a few degrees away from the vertical, and not at all to horizontal lines. There are a few broadly tuned channels for each dimension of the stimulus. Numbers are disputed but, for example, there may be three color, six size, and 18 orientation channels. To identify a specific stimulus, a comparison is made between the activity in two or more channels. Thus, stationary could be the percept resulting from equal excitement in movement channels tuned for motion to the left and the right.

There are several psychophysical methods to study channels. For example, if a subject views stimuli of one size, selective adaptation will occur. The subject will be less sensitive to stimuli of that size. Sensitivity to similar sizes will be reduced but not as much. Stimuli of very different sizes will be unaffected if selective adaptation to one size specifically has fatigued the channels sensitive to that size. The spread of adaptation to neighboring sizes gives an idea of the broadness of the tuning of the channel.

Stereopsis and other hyperacuities

Stereoscopic depth is another product of this stage in visual processing. Stereopsis is based on the geometry of vision. The two eyes look at the world from slightly different vantage points. This results in slight differences (or retinal disparities) between the two retinal images. These differences can be used as a clue to three-dimensional depth. Retinal disparities smaller than the diameter of a single photoreceptor can give rise to depth sensations. The ability to detect such small features is known as hyperacuity. There are several hyperacuities, all probably the result of computations in the visual cortex. One example is vernier acuity, the ability to detect an offset between two adjacent line segments. Offsets of 6 seconds of arc (60 minutes in a degree, and 60 seconds in a minute) can be detected. Normal visual acuity is about ten times coarser. The temporal analog of spatial acuity is critical flicker frequency (CFF). A light can be seen to vary over time if its rate of flicker is below the CFF of about 40–50 Hz.

Visual constancies

As important as the ability to extract features from the retinal image is the ability to ignore certain aspects. For example, large changes in illumination (e.g., from artificial light to sunlight) do not change the perceived color of objects even though very different wavelengths fall on the retina. This color constancy allows the observer to perceive invariant properties of objects independent of irrelevant changes in the retinal image. Other related constancies include those of brightness, shape, and size.

Visual inference

Following the analysis of the output of the broadly tuned channels, the visual system is able to identify the color, motion, depth, etc., of stimuli present at any spot in the image. Next, to determine what objects created the image, the visual system applies a set of rules to the representation it has generated. The set is large and by no means entirely known. It presumably includes rules such as "If A occludes part of B, then A is in front of B." Other rules would allow shape to be inferred from the pattern of shading or from motion, and so forth. Many visual illusions are the result of misapplication of these rules. For example, the ability to use shading to discover shape requires certain assumptions about how light forms shadows in the real world. In photographic negatives, the assumptions are violated and the perception of shape is severely impaired.

These rules and assumptions are applied automatically and are, in general, not accessible to conscious introspection by the observer. With unusual exceptions, the observer has no choice about the interpretation of the visual scene. Objects are perceived in various relationships to each other without apparent effort or apparent passage of time. When situations arise in which the interpretation of the visual scene is not effortless and instantaneous, the event is noteworthy. Examples include ambiguous figures such as those in the works of Escher.

The objects that have been found in the image now must be identified as cat, dog, friend, house, or whatever. Wide agreement does not exist on how this is accomplished. Consider the number of objects that can be identified as dogs. Dogs come in a vast range of sizes, shapes, and colors. Further, a single dog can form a huge number of different images on the retina depending on the animal's location relative to the observer. Nevertheless, like the rest of visual perception, the identification of an object usually is instantaneous and apparently effortless.

Visual development

The course of development of some basic visual functions has been traced. For example, visual acuity is poor at birth and steadily improves over the first two years of life. Color vision, by contrast, seems to be essentially normal at or near birth. Stereopsis develops automatically about three months after birth. The origin of the rules of perception is not entirely known. Clearly, some must be learned. We learn, for instance, what objects are to be identified as telephones. Others may well be innate. For example, do we learn the rule that states that occluding objects are in front of occluded objects, or does that rule come prewired in the visual system? We do not yet know.

Visual cognition

These highest levels of visual processing are not entirely independent of conscious intervention by the observer. While no amount of thinking will make a red region look blue, observer's expectations can influence the perceived identity of objects. A child who says a cloud looks like a duck or cow has brought object recognition under cognitive control, and such comments may alter a bystander's perception of that object. When stimuli are degraded, the control of perception by expectation may be particularly noticeable. Thus, on a dark night, "How easy a bush be supposed a bear."

Further reading

Introductory Text
Goldstein EB (1984): *Sensation and Perception*. Belmont, Calif: Wadsworth

Advanced Text
Kaufman L (1974): *Sight and Mind*. New York: Oxford University Press

Visual System, Organization

John Allman

In most animals the eyes are directed laterally and the visual field is nearly panoramic, which enables them to detect the approach of potential predators from nearly all directions. In a few animals such as primates, cats, and owls, the eyes are directed frontally, and the visual field is thus constricted. It has often been suggested that frontally directed eyes in primates provide these creatures with a large binocular field, thus enabling them to make stereoscopic depth judgments when leaping from branch to branch. However, many prodigious branch leapers such as squirrels have laterally directed eyes. An alternative explanation offered by M. Cartmill is that ancestral primates, like cats and owls, were visual predators. Indeed the living primates that most resemble ancestral primates, the tarsiers, are predators. As I have noted elsewhere, cats, owls, and tarsiers have more in common than just being predators; they are also nocturnal, and it is highly probable that ancestral primates were nocturnal as well. Because of bilateral symmetry, all predators tend to position themselves so their prey lie straight ahead of them when they prepare to strike. Thus the portion of the visual field straight ahead is particularly important to the predator as it observes the prey's defenses. The neural representations in the brain of the portion of the visual field straight ahead are commensurately expanded. However, in the dimly illuminated world of the nocturnal predator, the optical clarity of the retinal image also plays an important role. In the eye of the predator, as in most optical systems, the clearest image is created by the rays near the rotational axis of the system. Thus for an animal with laterally directed eyes the retinal image for objects straight ahead will be somewhat compromised. In a brightly illuminated environment this image degradation can be minimized by stopping down the pupil and thus restricting the off axial rays, but this option is not available to the nocturnal predator. Thus optimal retinal image quality for the portion of the visual field straight ahead would provide a selective advantage to nocturnal predators with frontally directed eyes. Frontally directed eyes offer several additional advantages to nocturnal predators. Binocular correlation of the retinal images might facilitate the detection of camouflaged prey, and binocular summation might facilitate the detection of prey under low light conditions.

Predatory primates use their hands to seize their prey. This behavior presumably is linked to the development of neural mechanisms for eye-hand coordination. The meticulous manual grooming of the fur, including the removal of minute ectoparasites, may be a relic in higher primates of the predatory behavior of earlier primates.

R.D. Martin has suggested that the ancestral primate adaption was to the "fine branch niche." Ancestral primates were small creatures who used their prehensile hands and feet to grasp the fine terminal branches of tropical trees, a niche rich in insect and small vertebrate prey. This is a particularly complex environment in which to move about since the fine branches provide an unstable platform, thus placing greater demands on the orienting functions of the visual system.

The fossils of Eocene primates more than 50 million years old possessed expanded bony orbits that in life encircled large eyes and cranial endocasts that reveal a commensurate expansion of the occipital and temporal lobes. The organization of the cerebral cortex in early primates cannot, of course, be determined directly, but it is possible to arrive at a number of inferences on the basis of what is known of the physiology and anatomy of the cortex in living primates. Figure 1 illustrates the organization of the cortex in the owl monkey. All the occipital, much of the temporal, and even some of the parietal and frontal lobes are devoted to the processing of visual input. There are nine visuotopically organized cortical areas, and there is partial evidence for several more in the posterior part of the temporal lobe. In addition there are extensive regions of inferotemporal, posterior parietal, and frontal eye field cortex that certainly are devoted to visual processing but that do not appear to contain orderly maps of the visual field. Evidence from macaque monkeys indicates a comparable array of visual areas in these primates as well. My collaborators and I have been mapping the organization of the visual cortex in a prosimian, galago, which contains the first visual area (V-I), the second visual area (V-II), the dorsolateral area (DL), the middle temporal area (MT), and additional areas that may correspond to the medial area (M) and the ventral posterior (VP) and ventral anterior (VA) ares. In the galago, the region corresponding to inferotemporal cortex appears to be visuotopically organized and may correspond to only the posterior portion of temporal cortex in simian primates. Since the last common ancestor of owl monkey and galagos lived no more recently than the Eocene and since there is fossil evidence for occipital and temporal lobe expansion in that period, it is likely that early primates possessed an extensive array of cortical areas including V-I, V-II, DL, MT, and probably several more.

The main source of visual input to the cerebral cortex arrives via the geniculostriate system which contains two principal ascending pathways originating in the retina. The first is a fast conducting pathway that is relayed by neurons in the magnocellular laminae of the lateral geniculate nucleus to layer 4C-alpha of V-I, then to layer 4B in V-I, then to MT. The neurons in layer 4B of V-I and in MT are usually highly sensitive to the direction of stimulus motion. Findings by J.A. Movshon and his collaborators show that some MT neurons respond to the apparent direction of motion of complex patterns, whereas V-I neurons respond to the actual direction of motion of the components of the stimulus, which can be quite different from the apparent direction of motion of the whole pattern. Thus the properties of MT neurons more nearly match perception and constitute a significant elaboration of function beyond that found in V-I.

F. Miezin, E. McGuinness, and I have found that the total receptive field (TRF) for most MT neurons is much larger than the classical receptive field (CRF) that is mapped with a single stimulus against a featureless background. As illustrated in Figure 2, we first mapped the CRF and determined its preferred direction to a pattern of moving dots. We then found that the second set of dots moving entirely outside the CRF profoundly and selectively influenced the response to stimuli presented simultaneously within the CRF. We also found that the velocity of movement in the surround influenced the response from the CRF (see Fig. 3). The detection of differential shearing motion by these neurons could be the basis of depth perception through motion parallax. The areas of the surrounds were 50 to 100 times that of the CRF and thus included much of the visual field. MT neurons thus make a simultaneous comparision between the direction and velocity of movement of objects occurring locally within their CRFs and globally over nearly the whole visual field. There is increasing evidence that neurons at many levels in the visual system make analogous local-global comparisons. The brain contains many maps of the visual field as revealed by the topographic organization of CRFs, but the TRFs for many neurons in these maps may extend throughout much of the visual field. The TRFs would provide mechanisms of local-global comparisons embedded in visuotopic matrices that may serve as the basis for many functions in vision, such as perceptual constancies and figure-ground discrimination.

The second major ascending pathway is slower conducting and is relayed from the retina by the neurons in the parvocellular laminae of the lateral geniculate nucleus to layer 4C-beta in V-I, then to layer 3 in V-I, then to V-II, then to DL, then to inferotemporal cortex. This system appears to be devoted in part to the analysis of form. S. Petersen, J. Baker, and I have found that DL neurons are highly selective to the size

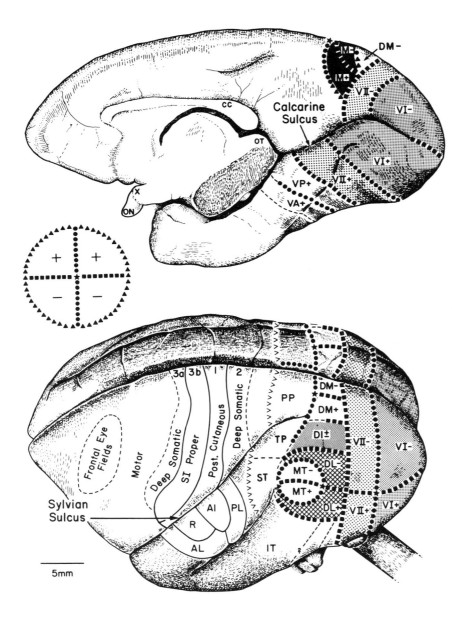

Figure 1. Representations of the sensory domains in the cerebral cortex of the owl monkey. Top, ventromedial view; bottom, a dorsolateral view. On the left is a perimeter chart of the visual field. Symbols in this chart are superimposed on the surface of the visual cortex. Pluses indicate upper-quadrant representations; minuses, lower quadrants; dashed lines, borders of areas that correspond to the representations of the relatively peripheral parts of the visual field, but not the extreme periphery. The row of Vs indicates the approximate border of visually responsive cortex. The dashed line broken by a question mark indicates an uncertain border. AI, first auditory area; AL, anterolateral auditory area; CC, corpus callosum; DI, dorsointermediate visual area; DL, dorsolateral visual area; DM, dorsomedial visual area; IT, inferotemporal visual cortex; M, medial visual area; MT, middle temporal visual area; ON, optic nerve; OT, optic tectum; PL, posterolateral auditory area; PP, posterior parietal visual cortex; R, rostral auditory area; VA, ventral anterior visual area; VP, ventral posterior visual area; X, optic chiasm. Reproduced from Allman JM, Baker JF, Newsome WT, Petersen SE (1981): Visual topography and function cortical visual areas in the owl monkey. In: *Multiple Visual Areas*, Woolsey CN, ed, with permission of Humana Press.

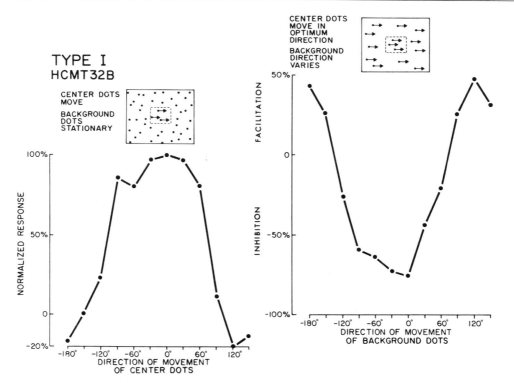

Figure 2. Direction-selective neuron with an antagonistic direction-selective surround recorded from the middle temporal visual area (MT) in an owl monkey. The left graph depicts the response of the cell to 12 directions of movement of an array of random dots within an area coextensive with its classical receptive field (CRF), the small dashed line rectangle. The response is normalized so that 0% is equal to the average level of spontaneous activity sampled for 2-second periods before each presentation. Negative percentages in the left graph indicate inhibition relative to spontaneous activity. In the left graph, the response to the optimum direction is 100%. The right graph depicts the response of the cell to different directions of background movement while the CRF was simulta-neously stimulated with an array of dots moving in the cell's preferred direction. In the right graph, the CRF was stimulated by the array moving in the optimum direction during the 2-second sample periods preceding background movement, and thus a response of 100% in the left graph is equivalent to 0% in the right graph. The stimulus conditions are depicted schematically above each graph. In the actual experiment, the dots were 50% dark, 50% light, and the background was much larger relative to the center than is depicted schematically. Reproduced from Allman J, Miezin F, McGuinness E (1985): Stimulus specific responses from beyond the classical receptive field. *Annu Rev Neurosci*, Cowan WM, ed, with permission of Annual Reviews, Inc.

and shape of visual stimuli irrespective of their exact position within the CRF. R. Desimone and collaborators have found striking evidence for shape selectivity for neurons in inferotemporal cortex. Infero-temporal cortex is also strongly implicated in the ability to learn to discriminate visual shapes. There is evidence in macaque monkeys that a distinct subsystem within this pathway may be devoted to the analysis of color. There are also ascending pathways from V-II to DM, M, and VP.

Why are there so many cortical visual areas? In attempting to develop computer analogs to visual perception, D. Marr enunciated the principle of modular design. Marr stated that any large computation should be broken down into a collection of small modules as independent as possible from one another. Otherwise, "the process as a whole becomes extremely difficult to debug or improve, whether by a human engineer or in the course of natural evolution, because a small change to improve one part has to be accompanied by many simultaneous changes elsewhere." The formation of modules may have been produced by the replication of visual areas in evolution. The replication of existing structures appears to have been a fundamental mechanism in evolution. The paleontologist W. Gregory proposed that a common mechanism of evolution is the replication of a body part due to a genetic mutation in a single

generation, which is then followed in subsequent generations by the gradual divergence of structure and functions of the duplicated parts. S. Ohno has theorized that duplicated genes escape the pressures of natural selection operating on the original gene and thereby can accumulate mutations that enable the replicated gene to encode for a novel protein capable of assuming new functions, and indeed there exist many examples of DNA sequence homologies in replicated genes. The same evolutionary advantages that hold for the replication of genes may also hold for the replication of visual areas.

Finally to return to the ecological and behavioral theme, the restricted visual field of animals with frontally directed eyes increases their vulnerability to attack. This limitation appears to have been compensated by good sound-localizing ability in owls, cats, and some prosimian primates. Another solution is to recruit extra sets of eyes by living in social groups. Thus the restricted visual field resulting from frontally directed eyes may have provided a selective pressure favoring the development of social organization in primates. In most mammals olfaction plays an important role in social communication. Olfactory cues define territorial boundaries and express sexual receptivity. The amygdala receives major olfactory input and is reciprocally connected with the neuroendocrine control centers of the hypothalamus, and thus is likely to mediate the

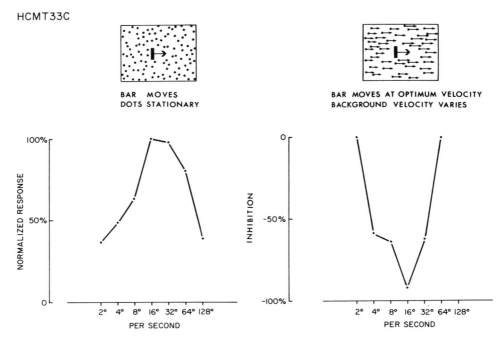

HCMT33C

Figure 3. The effect of center and background velocity on a neuron recorded from the middle temporal visual area (MT) in an owl monkey. The left graph is a velocity tuning curve for a bar moving in the preferred direction with a stationary random dot background. The right graph is a velocity tuning curve for background movement while simultaneously presenting the bar moving at the optimum velocity (16° per second).

Note the strong suppression of the response by movement in the surround at the preferred velocity for movement within the CRF. Reproduced from Allman J, Miezin F, McGuinness E (1985): Stimulus specific responses from beyond the classical receptive field. In: *Annu Rev Neurosci* Cowan WM, ed, with permission of Annual Reviews, Inc.

linkage between olfactory cues and behavior. In higher primates, the olfactory system is much reduced and the amygdala receives its main sensory input from the neocortex, particularly from the highest levels of visual and auditory processing in the temporal cortex. Portions of the amygdala also project back onto the border between layers 1 and 2 in cortical visual areas. These connections may activate long-term memory processes in the neocortex. There is a positive correlation in primate species between the amount of neocortex relative to body weight and the size and complexity of the species' social groups. In higher primates, social communication is mediated largely through visual and acoustic channels, which have much greater information-carrying capacities than olfactory cues. Neurons in the depths of the superior temporal sulcus in monkeys are selectively responsive to faces, and neurons in the amygdala respond selectively to particular facial expressions. Thus during the course of primate evolution there has been a transformation of social communication from pheromones and olfaction to facial expression and vision.

Further reading

Allman JM (1977): Evolution of the visual system in the early primates. In: *Progress of Psychobiology and Physiological Psychology*, Sprague JM, Epstein AN, eds, 7:1–53. New York: Academic

Allman JM, Miezin F, McGuinness E (1985): Stimulus specific responses from beyond the classical receptive field: Neurophysiological mechanisms for local-global comparisons in visual neurons. In: *Annu Rev Neurosci* Cowan WM et al, eds, 8:407–430. Palo Alto: Annual Reviews

Amaral DG, Price JL (1984): Amygdalo-cortical projections in the monkey (*Macaca fascicularis*). *J Comp Neurol* 230:465–496

Desimone R, Albright TD, Gross CG, Bruce C (1984): Stimulus-selective properties of interior temporal neurons in the macaque. *J Neurosci* 4:2051–2062

Marr D (1976): Early processing of visual information. *Phil Trans R Soc Lond* B275:483–519

Movshon JA, Adelson EH, Gizzi MS, Newsome WT (1986): The analysis of moving visual patterns. *Exp Brain Res,* in press

Stephan H, Andy OJ (1970): The allocortex in primates. In: *The Primate Brain*, Noback CR, Montagna W, eds New York: Appleton

Visual System, Siamese Cats

Carla J. Shatz

In Siamese cats, a genetic mutation at the albino locus, known for producing the characteristic Siamese coat color, also somehow causes an excessive number of ganglion cell axons from each retina to cross in the optic chiasm and travel to the wrong side of the brain. As a consequence, the central visual pathways of Siamese cats are abnormal; abnormalities are also found behaviorally and in eye movement control, since these animals demonstrate a marked strabismus. Thus, the Siamese mutation provides a unique opportunity to study how the visual system responds to abnormal inputs from the two eyes. And because a gene rather than a scalpel is responsible, it should be possible to learn about some of the cellular and molecular events that control the routing of optic axons in mammals.

The chiasmatic misrouting of ganglion cell axons provides target nuclei, such as the lateral geniculate nucleus (LGN) in the thalamus with an abnormally large contribution from the contralateral retina and a correspondingly diminished one from the ipsilateral retina. In order to identify the population of ganglion cells responsible for this increased contralateral pro-

jection, tracers such as horseradish peroxidase (HRP) have been injected into the LGN to label ganglion cells by means of retrograde transport. When this experiment is performed in normally pigmented animals, results show that the vast majority of ganglion cells projecting to the contralateral LGN are situated in the nasal retina (see Fig. 1A). Consequently, a very sharp line, called the line of decussation or nasotemporal division, subdivides the retina into contralaterally (nasal retina) and ipsilaterally (temporal retina) projecting ganglion cell populations.

In Siamese cats, similar experiments show that, as in normally pigmented cats, ganglion cells in the nasal retina send their axons across the chiasm to terminate in the opposite LGN. In addition, however, many ganglion cells in the temporal retina also send their axons across the chiasm, as shown in Figure 1B. Others make a normal uncrossed projection to the LGN on the same side. As a consequence, since the temporal retina contains a mixture of abnormal contralaterally projecting and normal ipsilaterally projecting ganglion cells, a normal sharp line of decussation is not present in Siamese cats.

The retinal ganglion cell population in the cat, as in most vertebrates, is not homogeneous but rather is composed of several functionally and morphologically distinct subclasses. Three major classes have been defined on the basis of soma size: alpha, large; beta, medium; gamma, small. Studies suggest that the effect of the Siamese mutation may not be expressed evenly on all classes, since it appears that a disproportionally large number of the misprojecting ganglion cells from temporal retina are alpha cells.

The thalamic abnormality

In normally pigmented animals, the lateral geniculate nucleus receives projections from ganglion cells of the nasal retina of the contralateral eye and the temporal retina of the ipsilateral eye. These projections terminate in separate LGN layers, with axons from the contralateral eye going to layers A, C, and C2, and those from the ipsilateral eye to layers A1 and C1, as shown in Figure 1A. In Siamese cats the contralateral projection from the nasal retina terminates as usual in layers A and C (see Fig. 1B). The projection from the temporal retina also terminates as usual in layers A1 and C1, the difference being that in Siamese cats most of the projection to these layers now comes from the contralateral eye (compare Figs. 1A and 1B). As a consequence, layer A1 in Siamese cats is broken up into a large zone that receives abnormal input from the temporal retina of the contralateral eye (Fig. 1B: abnormal segment of layer A1 = AbA1) and smaller medial and lateral islands receiving what is left of the normal temporal retinal projection from the ipsilateral eye (Fig. 1B: medial normal

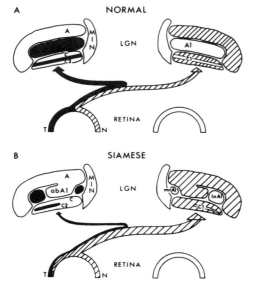

Figure 1. Diagram of the retinogeniculate projection in normally pigmented (A) and Siamese (B) cats. Hatched areas indicate zones of contralaterally projecting retinal ganglion cells and their sites of termination within LGN. Black areas indicate zones of ipsilaterally projecting ganglion cells. T, temporal retina; N, nasal retina. See text for further details. Reprinted by permission from *Nature*, 300:525–529, Copyright © 1982 Macmillan Journals Limited.

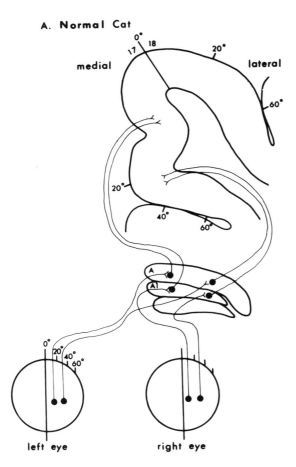

A. Normal Cat

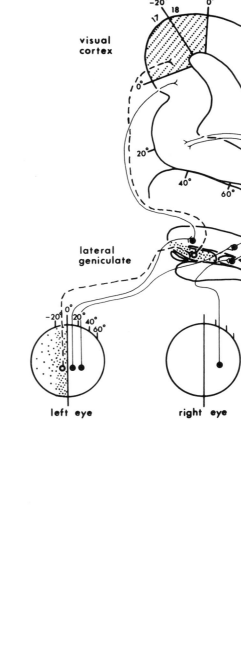

B. Boston Siamese

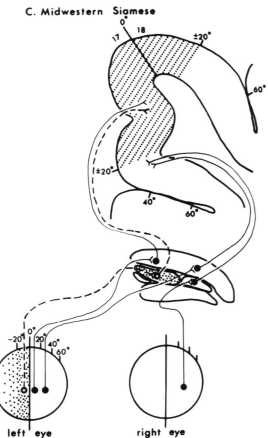

C. Midwestern Siamese

Figure 2. Diagram showing pathways from the retina to cortex in normal (A), Boston (B), and Midwestern (C) Siamese cats. In Siamese cats, abnormal projections are shown by dashed lines, and the participating abnormal regions within the retina, LGN, and cortex that represent roughly the first 20 degrees of ipsilateral visual field are stippled. For simplicity, only connections between the right LGN and cortex have been indicated, and connections to the C laminae and the medial normal segment of lamina A1 in the LGN have been omitted. See text for further details.

segment of layer A1 = mNA1; lateral normal segment of layer A1 = 1NA1).

In Siamese cats, the projection from the retina to the LGN is systematic but substantially different from that present in normally pigmented cats. In normal animals, microelectrode recordings have shown that each LGN receives information about the contralateral half of the visual field from both eyes. This comes about because retinal ganglion cells from the nasal retina of one eye and the temporal retina of the other eye both represent points in the contralateral half of the visual field (Fig. 2A). Consequently, each LGN layer contains an orderly map of the contralateral visual field from one eye or the other. In Siamese cats, in contrast, the LGN receives information about both ipsilateral and contralateral visual fields, but only from one (contralateral) eye (Fig. 2B,C). The input is still topographically organized, with layer A containing an orderly map of the contralateral visual field, and the abnormal segment of layer A1 containing an orderly map of up to 20 degrees or more of the ipsilateral visual field.

The cortical abnormality

The primary visual cortex (area 17) deals with the abnormal representation of the ipsilateral visual field in the Siamese cat LGN in two different ways. In the first, the projection of LGN neurons to the primary visual cortex is similar in pattern to that seen in normally pigmented cats. As shown in Figure 2A, in normal animals, LGN cells at corresponding positions in layers A and A1 send their axons to the same location within visual cortex. Since visual field coordinates in the two layers are identical, this geniculocortical projection pattern ensures that visual field coordinates are precisely aligned and topographically ordered at the cortical level. However, in Siamese cats (Fig. 2C), this anatomical arrangement has the bizarre result of conferring onto each cortical location the representation of two mirror-symmetric visual field positions: one in the normal contralateral hemifield and the other in the abnormal ipsilateral hemifield. This pattern is called the Midwestern projection pattern because it was first observed in Siamese cats by J. Kaas and R. Guillery (1973) in Wisconsin.

Physiological mapping experiments in 1971 by D. Hubel and T. Wiesel have demonstrated that an entirely different projection pattern can be found in Siamese cats as well: the Boston projection pattern (Fig. 2B). Here, the abnormal geniculate regions representing the ipsilateral visual field (e.g., the abnormal segment of layer A1) now project to their own strip of cortex, which is separate but adjacent to that receiving normal input from geniculate layers representing the contralateral visual field. Recent physiological experiments suggest that both patterns can sometimes be found in the same animal in different parts of the visual cortex (the Boston pattern in these cases was always found in cortical regions representing the inferior visual fields).

It should be emphasized that the Boston pattern represents an extensive and orderly anatomical reorganization of the geniculocortical projection, and therefore can be readily distinguished from the Midwestern pattern by anatomical methods. Thus, in Boston Siamese cats the 17/18 border receives input only from LGN neurons situated at the lateral edge of the abnormal segment of layer A1, whereas in Midwestern Siamese cats neurons in the medial sectors of both layers A and A1 project to the 17/18 border.

Animals with the Boston projection pattern can also be distinguished from their Midwestern counterparts by behavioral criteria. Visual field testing of Siamese cats, in conjunction with anatomical studies, have shown that Midwestern Siamese

cats suffer from blindness in their nasal visual fields (temporal retinas) when tested monocularly. Of course, it is not known how this blindness arises, but it is noteworthy that in microelectrode recordings from the primary visual cortex of Midwestern cats neurons driven from the ipsilateral visual field (temporal retina) were rarely encountered. Thus Guillery has proposed that the pathway from temporal retina to visual cortex is somehow ineffective in influencing cortical cells—hence the suppression seen behaviorally in Midwestern cats.

The callosal abnormality

The unusual reorganization of the geniculocortical projection seen in Boston Siamese cats has further consequences for higher order visual connections, in particular, those subserved by the corpus callosum. In normally pigmented animals anatomical and physiological experiments have shown that callosal connections between areas 17 in the two hemispheres link up visuotopically similar zones. Since the only visual field coordinates common to the two hemispheres are those near the vertical midline, only the circumscribed zones near the 17/18 border are interconnected with each other via the corpus callosum (Fig. 3A).

The same anatomical pattern of interhemispheric connections in Boston Siamese cats would be of little use functionally since cells receiving input from mirror-symmetric visual field coordinates ($+20°$ and $-20°$) would be connected together. In fact, these connections are not found in adult Boston Siamese cats. Instead, the pattern of callosal connections has

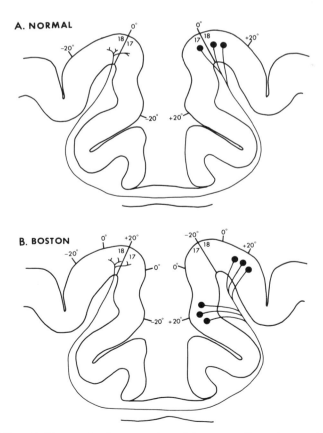

Figure 3. Diagram showing connections of the corpus callosum in normal and Boston Siamese cats.

undergone a remarkable reorganization (Fig. 3B) so that appropriate visuotopic relations are preserved despite altered connectivity. For example, cells at the 17/18 border in one hemisphere are now connected to cells deep within areas 17 and 18 in the opposite hemisphere that receive input from the same visual field coordinates. Furthermore, since both hemispheres share a good deal of the visuotopic map (up to 20° to either side of the vertical midline of the visual field), broad regions of areas 17 and 18 are interconnected by the corpus callosum in these animals.

The ability of cortical neurons in Boston Siamese cats to establish connections with appropriate counterparts elsewhere that carry similar visuotopic information is not restricted to the corpus callosum. Another example is in the recurrent projection from cortex back to LGN. In the Boston variety, neurons at the 17/18 border project only to the lateral tip of the abnormal segment of layer A1; there is no projection to layer A. In other words, cells representing the same visual field coordinates (about 15–20· into the ipsilateral visual field) within LGN and cortex are reciprocally interconnected. In contrast, in Midwestern cats, as in normally pigmented ones, both layers A and A1 of the LGN receive projections from cortical cells at the 17/18 border.

The remarkable preservation of appropriate topographic relationships in Boston Siamese cats seen in callosal and corticogeniculate connections may not be present in corticocortical connections within the same hemisphere. For example, cells at the 17/18 border send projections to zones deep within areas 17 and 18 on the same side of the brain; these, then, are entirely novel connections not seen in normal animals that link neurons subserving mirror-symmetric visual field coordinates.

The systematic rearrangements found in the connections of geniculocortical, callosal, corticogeniculate and even corticocortical pathways in the Boston variety of Siamese cat suggest that the basic patterns of connectivity in these pathways are not immutable. On the contrary, these pathways are susceptible to modification, especially in order to permit appropriate visuotopic relations. Exactly how visuotopically appropriate connections are established in these animals is unknown, but it is likely that visual experience plays an important role.

Mechanism of Siamese gene action

Although very little is known about the exact relationship between the Siamese gene (an allele at the albino locus) and the chiasmatic misrouting of ganglion cell axons, a good deal of accumulated circumstantial evidence suggests that the primary site of gene action is peripheral to the optic chiasm. Perhaps most compelling is the observation that chiasm misrouting occurs in almost every mammal in which there is a reduction in pigment level within the retinal pigment epithelium. During normal fetal development, the optic stalk is also transiently pigmented, but in Siamese cats and other species with pigment abnormalities, the amount of pigment within the optic stalk is severely reduced. These observations have led several researchers to suggest that pigment or a related gene product may be required for the normal positioning of ganglion cell axons within the optic nerve, and position in turn may determine the chiasmatic fate of axons. Consistent with this hypothesis is the observation that during fetal development in Siamese cats, ganglion cell axons cross at the chiasm in abnormally large numbers at the outset.

In view of these considerations, the reorganization of central visual pathways seen in Boston Siamese cats is likely to be a secondary effect of the misrouting: ganglion cell axons are rerouted, thereby confronting the rest of the brain with abnormal input from the periphery. Thus the cascade-like rewiring of central visual connections found in Boston Siamese cats suggests that during development, retinal input can play an essential role in determining the pattern of central connections in the visual system.

Further reading

Cooper ML, Pettigrew JD (1979): The retinothalamic pathways in Siamese cats. *J Comp Neurol* 187:313–348

Hubel DH, Wiesel TN (1971): Aberrant visual projections in the Siamese cat. *J Physiol (Lond)* 218:33–62

Kaas JH, Guillery RW (1973): The transfer of abnormal visual field representations from the dorsal lateral geniculate nucleus to the visual cortex in Siamese cats. *Brain Res* 59:61–95

Shatz CJ (1979): Abnormal connections in the visual system of Siamese cats. *Soc Neurosci Symp* 4:121–141

Shatz CJ, Kliot M (1982): Prenatal misrouting of the retinogeniculate pathway in Siamese cats. *Nature* 300:525–529

Silver J (1984): Studies on the factors that govern directionality of axonal growth in the embryonic optic nerve and at the optic chiasm of mice. *J Comp Neurol* 223:238–251

Strongin AC, Guillery RW (1981): The distribution of melanin in the developing optic stalk and its relation to cellular degeneration. *J Neurosci* 1:1193–1204

Visual System Development, Invertebrates

Eduardo R. Macagno and Ian A. Meinertzhagen

The visual systems of most invertebrate groups arise following the outgrowth of axons from photoreceptors which develop from the ectodermal epithelium independently of the nerve centers which they innervate; peripherally derived visual interneurons are exceptional. This is in contrast to vertebrates where the retina forms from an embryological outgrowth of the forebrain, with several classes of interneurons. Most studies on invertebrates are descriptive and preferentially treat eye development. Few studies are analytical and fewer treat the visual centers. Yet the topographic ordering, the small numbers of their identifiable neurons, and the many other model characteristics of invertebrate neuropils especially recommend these centers for studies in neural development and regeneration, notably the compound eyes of arthropods and the highly developed single-lens eyes of certain molluscs. Modern studies have tended to canonize selected species (especially the flies *Drosophila* and *Musca,* and the water-flea *Daphnia*) to the unwarranted neglect of other equally deserving groups—cephalopods, pectinid scallops, spiders, and salps to name but a few. A comprehensive review by Meinertzhagen and Macagno is forthcoming.

Eye development

Most invertebrate eyes arise from the ectodermal epithelium in one of two main ways. The first is by the formation of a fold and invagination to create a pit, open to the outside, or a vesicle that subsequently becomes internalized. The second, delamination, is by the thickening of a region as cells divide, grow, and differentiate, followed by the formation of the layers that form the retina. These can either remain as part of the epithelium or detach and move interiorly into the body cavity. The topography of the epithelium is conserved in the retinal layer of photoreceptors following invagination and delamination in situ, whereas it must be reconstituted secondarily following the inward migration of epithelial surface cells. Different animal groups may use different modes of eye development, but in some, both developmental origins are described, even in the different eyes of a single species.

The flagellate protozoans *Erythropsis* and *Warnowia* have elaborate ocellar organelles with a dioptric hyalosome and pigmentary melanosome. These two components dissociate and duplicate during cell division, the daughter organelles recombining afterward. In Cnidaria, the ocellus of the medusa of *Cladonema* arises from an ectodermal primordium from which differentiate photoreceptor, corneal, and pigment cells, the lens arising in the latter. In turbellarians with direct development, eyespots appear in the ectoderm and then sink into the mesoderm, enlarge, and divide to provide multiple pairs. In annelids, eyes are usually simple eyecup ocelli frequently with one or few photoreceptors that arise, in prostomial eye-

cups in leeches, from epidermal thickenings. Only in errant polychaetes are elaborate eyes found, which are variably said to arise either from the epidermis without invagination, or by delamination from an anlage, apparently of ectodermal origin, lying between ectoderm and pharynx and containing a special cell which secretes the lens. Differentiation occurs in a wave—first in the inner, retinal layer. By contrast, the pair of ocelli in Onycophora arises by invagination from an epidermal placode, which pinches off to form a vesicle lined with everted microvillar photoreceptors. Echinoderms have multiple simple ocelli on optic cushions, and these form following the invagination of relatively few cells from the epidermis. Among the various prevertebrate chordate groups, interesting eyes are found in salps, which have a single, dorsal eye pushed out in vertebrate fashion from a crescentic optic ridge of the cerebral ganglion to form an ocular disc. In the asexual chain form of the life cycle, the ocular disc folds up, turns over, and produces a layer of inverted photoreceptors abutting a layer of everted ones and then an everted secondary eye.

Clear accounts of eye development are generally restricted to groups with elaborate eyes, especially arthropods and molluscs. Large, single-lens cephalic eyes of gastropod and cephalopod molluscs, which project directly to the brain, generally arise by invagination of an ectodermal placode either de novo or during regeneration (*Strombus, Cardium, Helix,* etc.); details vary depending on whether development is direct or via a veliger larva and on the complexity of nonneural ocular components. Mantle eyes in bivalves have diverse origins and include both single-lens eyes and the compound eyes in arcid clams. In *Pecten* they arise by delamination of an epithelial placode secondarily reconstituted after migration from the epidermis. All show spectacular regenerative capabilities. Arthropods generally have ocelli that arise by invagination, delamination, or both in some insect groups. Spiders have single-lens frontal eyes that arise by invagination and lateral eyes that form by delamination. By contrast, compound eyes form by basically similar means in all groups, by delamination in situ from an embryonic epidermal placode internalized in holometabolous insects within imaginal discs borne in a postembryonic larva. In all other groups the eye generated in the embryo is augmented by ommatidial increments added during the intermolts. In diplopod myriapods ocelli are produced by individual anlagen and accumulate with each molt, in rows, reminiscent of ommatidial additions in hemimetabolous insects.

Photoreceptor morphogenesis also illustrates a basic dichotomy, despite diversity in many of its details within different groups. Following delamination, photoreceptors are usually oriented with their axons arising basally and their photoreceptive organelles·distally with respect to the path and direction of light entry (the everted type). In invaginated eyes photoreceptor orientation is variable, sometimes having axons which exit through the base of the eye or through the apical opening of the eyecup (the inverted type). Numerous exceptions exist, and the transition between inverted and everted types is apparently readily accomplished in evolutionary development. Spiders, for example, have principal eyes with everted photoreceptors formed following invagination and secondary eyes with inverted photoreceptors formed following delamination; certain species have converted photoreceptors (secondarily inverted photoreceptors produced within the principal eye). Invertebrates have both ciliary and rhabdomeric photoreceptors, even in some cases (e.g., *Pecten*) both in one eye, but no clear consensus has emerged for the phylogenetic development of the two types following Eakin's early formulation of an exclusive dichotomy between a protostomatous rhabdomeric and a deuterostomatous ciliary line of evolution. Various examples are now known in the development of rhabdomeric photoreceptors (which bear visual pigment upon microvilli) for the transient appearance of ciliary structures.

The pattern of eye growth is known best in arthropod compound eyes, which arise from epithelial cells of the head epidermis, either in a single wave (holometabolous insects, some Crustacea), or (all others) in an interrupted wave contributing a succession of strips laid at the anterior margin of the eye, one each between molts. Regional specializations of the eye (e.g., foveas in dragonflies or mantids) must therefore shift in the visual field with each molt, or be successively reconstructed. Generally, intermolt growth in eye size is mostly due to increased cell number, with lesser contributions from increases in size among existing cells, but species differ. The anterior eye margin in hemimetabolous insects is best thought of as a budding zone, perhaps harboring ommatidial stem cells. Ommatidial rudiments are laid down in the wake of a double posteroanterior wave of mitoses (*Drosophila, Ephestia*) which possibly overlap each other in the single wave of mitoses seen in the dragonfly. In *Drosophila* the two waves generate different cellular progeny, R1,6,7 in the posterior wave and the remainder in the anterior wave. The clonal progenies scatter in a band several ommatidia wide, and no clear lineage relationship exists between the photoreceptors of an ommatidium. It is presumed, by exclusion, that cell phenotype is determined epigenetically, by position within the ommatidial cluster. The sequence of cell clustering to form ommatidia in *Drosophila* is: first R8, to which are added R2 and 5 (giving a cluster with one line of symmetry), R3, 4 and then R1, 6 (with two lines of symmetry) and, last, R7 (giving an asymmetry).

Development of visual centers

Development of the optic lobe is described most clearly in arthropods. Ommatidia project upon the underlying optic neuropils with effectively perfect retinotopic precision (Fig. 1a). The effects of eye rotation experiments in locusts indicate the impartiality of ingrowing receptor axons for the particular cartridge in which they locate. Visual interneurons are the progeny of neuroblasts lying in two groups, the outer and inner optic anlagen, which generate the lamina and distal medulla, and the remaining medulla and lobula, respectively, in insects (Fig. 2C). In Crustacea the counterpart of an outer optic anlage only has so far been described (Fig. 2A,B); in the water-flea *Daphnia* this is the sole so-called optic lobe primordium. Ganglion cells in the outer optic neuropils are generated in mitotic waves which match those of the overlying receptor cells. Waves of cell death also occur. The numbers of dying cells are decreased in the dragonfly when the optic lobe is hyperinnervated by extra retina. Apparently cells are initially overproduced, most are commissioned by incoming

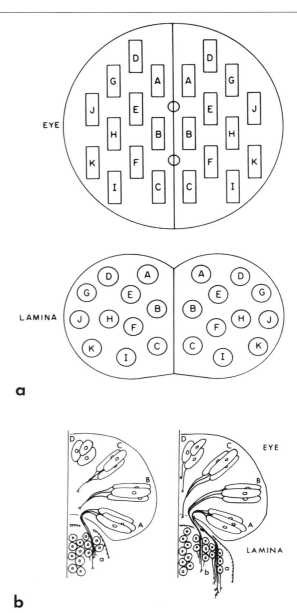

Figure 1. a. Schematic diagram of the compound eye (above) and optic lamina (below) in *Daphnia*, showing the locations of the individual ommatidia and the optic cartridges to which the photoreceptors of each ommatidium project. Both are viewed in a transverse projection, dorsal side up. Each lettered rectangle in the eye represents an ommatidium, and each similarly lettered circle in the lamina represents the corresponding optic cartridge. The projection is direct, without a chiasma. **b.** Schematic representation of the development of the eye-lamina projection in *Daphnia* at an early stage in its development (left) and several hours later (right). Only the right halves of the eye and lamina are depicted, in a view perpendicular to that shown in panel a. A, B, C, and D represent rows of ommatidia, each row at a different level of development; a and b represent forming optic cartridges. At both stages of development illustrated A, the most lateral ommatidia, are also the most developed, while D, the most medial, the least so. In the left panel, the axons from A have grown along the midline glial bridge that connects the eye and laminar anlage and have reached the target region, where they have begun to recruit laminar neurons, thus forming cartridge a. In the right panel, the axons from B have followed the same route as those of A and have completed the recruitment of five laminar neurons and formed cartridge b, displacing cartridge a laterally. Axons from C and D will subsequently repeat this process until the projection is completed.

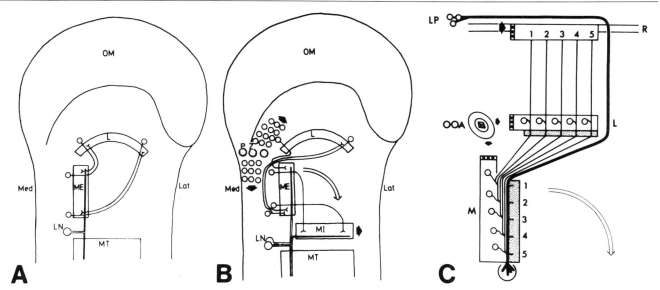

Figure 2. A–C. The assembly sequence of neuropil layers and of the fiber projections between them in the optic lobes of A, nonmalacostracan, and B, malacostracan Crustacea, and of C, a dipterous insect (fly). In all three examples, a common neuroblast population, the outer proliferation zone (PZ) or optic anlage (OOA), generates cells in two antiparallel directions. These assemble the cell cortices of lamina (L) and medulla (M) (in Crustacea: medulla externa, ME) in chronotopic sequence, like a conveyor belt. Following their birth, cells are continuously displaced from their anlage to await innervation from the overlying ommatidia (OM). Although not necessarily evolutionary homologs, the two neuropils—lamina and medulla—have major structural and developmental similarities in Crustacea and insects and grow identical chiasmal interconnecting pathways in malacostracan Crustacea and insects. In nonmalacostracans the axons of cell bodies in the lamina cortex penetrate the lamina and enter the medulla from its neuropil face, thus traversing directly between corre-

sponding neuropil faces. In Malacostraca and insects, on the other hand, a chiasma arises because the corresponding axons enter the medulla from the opposite direction, through its cortex, and in doing so invert their sequence. In the fly these axons grow along the path of Bolwig's nerve which originates in a rostral group of larval photoreceptors (LP). The chiasma appears more clearly in B and C when the medulla rotates its position with subsequent growth, in the direction shown by the open arrows. In A and B, tangential neurons (LN) from the medulla terminalis (MT) grow across the neuropil of the medulla externa and interna (MI), advancing to contact newly grown retinal innervation and the higher-order perpendicular pathways upon which it projects. Similar sequences occur in the optic lobe of insects. A and B after Elofsson and Dahl (1970), reprinted with permission of authors and Springer-Verlag. C after Meinertzhagen (1977), reprinted with permission of author and the Society for Neuroscience.

retinal innervation, but the remainder die. In two mutants of *Drosophila* cell death is dramatically increased. Receptor cell axons innervate new ganglion cells so produced, in successive rows corresponding to the wavefront of retinal differentiation. The cells that are newly innervated have been shown in *Daphnia* to be invariably newly postmitotic. Ingrowing receptor axons recruit ganglion cell bodies in the lamina in final groups of five. Each soma displays a stereotypic envelopment response in which it enwraps and forms transient gap junctions with the contacting receptor axons. The response is described in *Daphnia* but is possibly much more widespread. It appears in all cells contacted and in the same sequence in which they are contacted, but does not appear in cells from which retinal innervation is withheld and is delayed in cells to which that innervation arrives late. It thus manifests an inductive signal following which each cell is triggered to commence differentiation and spin out a neurite, growing along that of the retinal axon bundle in a secondary cascade.

The growth of axonal pathways is highly structured. Photoreceptor axons grow in centrally to innervate the lamina and distal medulla in a succession that reflects the ordered spatiotemporal sequence of retinal differentiation. Outgrowth within an ommatidial axon bundle is asynchronous. In the ommatidia of *Daphnia*, the axon from one of the photoreceptors (R1) has a well-defined growth cone and is the first to grow and contact target cells. Axons of other cells follow this lead axon, as illustrated in Figure 1b, and have much reduced growth cones or none. When the cell body of R1 is laser-deleted the

axon of another cell body takes over the role of the lead fiber, indicating the equivalence of the cells. In *Drosophila*, axon outgrowth occurs in an initial group of five, presumed those of R2–5,8, later supplemented by the remaining three. In many insect groups receptor axons grow postembryonically, centrally along the pathway provided by larval or nymphal visual systems, e.g., Bolwig's larval photoreceptor nerve in flies, larval ocelli in mosquitoes, stemmatal nerves in Lepidoptera and Coleoptera. Adult visual centers are then assembled around larval ones. These larval photoreceptor axons and the imaginal axons in other groups grow in the embryo, the first axons thus growing over very short distances to reach their target neurons, but elongating dramatically with subsequent growth, by towing. The first axons growing in *Daphnia* conform to the latter pattern, growing over a glial substrate. In these cases axon bundles growing later follow a preexisting neural pathway to the center, building up the fiber tract in which they grow and, at the same time, providing the substrate for yet further growth. The possible role of first-grown axons as uniquely essential pioneers for further axon growth has yet to be rigorously analyzed experimentally in insects. The sequence by which new axon bundles accrue to fiber tracts of old, and their relative positions within the tract confer the polarity of the resultant topographic map. Chiasmata form when this polarity inverts, as explained in Figures 2A–C. This occurs in the external chiasma of insects and malacostracan Crustacea. Many arachnid groups also have chiasmata.

In the fly, photoreceptor axons penetrate the lamina as part of their ommatidial axon bundle, then form expanded growth cones and gradually draw away from their parent bundle, with filopodia continuously exploring from the leading edge until the first set of neighboring monopolar cells is reached, whereupon each grows centripetally to form a terminal.

, Synaptogenesis follows the morphogenesis of terminals, as postsynaptic neurites contact presynaptic sites. In the fly, *Musca*, starting with L1 or L2, dendrites contact the photoreceptor terminal, each synaptic contact selectively accumulating other postsynaptic elements to make a tetrad; up to 50% of all contacts formed are lost. Although synaptic transmission can occur early, before all contacts are established, photoreceptors generate only slow responses of small amplitude, even to light far brighter than that to which they may normally be exposed.

Functional plasticity is shown by the visual system of bees and is being sought more widely. Bees reared in ultraviolet light have selectively reduced sensitivity to longer wavelengths in which they were deprived and selectively reduced (ca. 50%) frequencies of synaptic contacts on the terminals of green-sensitive photoreceptors. Central optic lobe neurons sprout following congenital deprivation of their visual inputs induced by laser-deletion in *Musca*, or by genetic mutation in *Drosophila*.

The morphogenetic interdependence of eye and visual centers has been revealed in cases where the development of one has been studied following the careful removal of the other. Some dependence of development in the visual centers upon innervation from the eye is generally found but quantitatively variable, whereas eye development is usually autonomous. In *Drosophila*, clones of mutant tissue with deranged cellular organization generated independently in the eye or optic lobe indicate most clearly that abnormal pattern is communicated from the retina to the lamina, but not in the opposite direction, findings which rigorously confirm the effects of deafferentation in many species. More central neuropils are volumetrically less affected by deafferentation. In congenitally eyeless mutant *Drosophila*, second-order neurons in the lamina never differentiate, but some neurons of the medulla do grow axons, albeit with abnormal morphogenesis. A qualitatively similar result follows deletions in the embryonic eye of *Daphnia*. Differentiation in the fly's lamina and medulla is largely unaffected by the absence of target cells in the lobula, indicating the relative absence of retrograde influences of central visual neuropils upon distal ones.

Further reading

Ali MA, ed (1984): *Photoreception and Vision in Invertebrates*. New York: Plenum Press, NATO ASI vol 74

Macagno ER (1984): Formation of ordered connections in the visual system of *Daphnia magna. Bioscience* 34:308–312

Meinertzhagen IA, Macagno ER (1987): Development of invertebrate visual systems. In: *Handbook of Physiology: Developmental Neurobiology* Edwards JS, Cowan WM, eds. Washington DC: American Physiological Society, in press

Meinertzhagen, I.A. (1973): Development of the compound eye and optic lobe of insects. In: *Developmental Neurobiology of Arthropods* Young D, ed. Cambridge: University Press

Westfall JA, ed (1982): *Visual Cells in Evolution*. New York: Raven Press

Visual System Development, Plasticity

Paul Grobstein and Kao Liang Chow

In research on visual system development, as elsewhere, the concept of plasticity has meant different things to different people at different times, and it is unlikely that the evolution of the meaning of the term is over. Any attempt at definition must thus take into account the plasticity of "plasticity." In speaking broadly of 20th century neurobiology, it is useful to distinguish three roughly successive periods. During the earliest phase, a major concern of investigators was with the issue of whether the adaptive organization of the visual system reflects predesign based on genetic information, as opposed to processes of adaptive shaping based on functional effectiveness. Plasticity was used to characterize the latter alternative and was understood to mean "the capacity to adjust functional organization based on sensory experience." In subsequent years, attention shifted to documenting the existence of orderly patterns of anatomical connections in the visual pathways and to the hypothesis that these resulted from a refined capacity of outgrowing axons to recognize and distinguish between target neurons based on cytochemical affinities. During this period, plasticity became more specifically linked to problems of anatomical connectivity but largely lost its reference to the broader problem of accounting for functionally appropriate organization. The term was generally used to refer to any phenomenon suggesting a capacity to make a pattern of connections other than the "normal" one, hence challenging the chemoaffinity hypothesis.

In recent years, it has become increasingly clear that the anatomical organization of the visual system is a good deal more fluid than had previously been suspected, that connection patterns may differ at different times during an individual lifetime and may be adjusted to fit different functional requirements. One needs to account not for a normal connection pattern but rather for the existence of the particular pattern appropriate for the functional demands at a given time. In this context, plasticity has begun to regain some of its earlier meaning. At the same time, current usage differs from that in the first phase, and borrows from that in the second, in that influences of sensory experience are no longer regarded as the sole mechanism by which functionally appropriate adjustments can occur. Many of the phenomena lumped together under plasticity during the second period are proving to reflect the existence of other mechanisms of adaptive adjustment. At the present time, visual system plasticity is probably best understood as the capability to make functionally appropriate adjustments in the anatomical connection patterns that make up the visual pathways.

The first phase: Functional organization, sensory experience, connectivity, and recognition

With the onset of active research on brain organization, it was natural that long-standing curiosities about the relative significances of innate and environmental influences on perception would begin to be posed in terms of the ontogeny of brain function and structure. Indeed, as early as 1892, H.H. Donaldson reported abnormalities in cortical thickness in the brain of a woman, Laura Bridgeman, blinded at a young age by scarlet fever. Bridgeman had lost vision in one eye several years before losing it in the other. Donaldson noted that the occipital cortex opposite her earlier blinded eye was thinner than that opposite the other eye and concluded that it was specifically visual deprivation that resulted in poor cortical development. What was unfortunately not clearly recognized at the time is that each eye sends signals to both visual cortices, a reality that significantly weakens Donaldson's conclusions. While studies of brain structure and sensory deprivation in the early part of the 20th century proved to be of marginal importance for subsequent research, a clinical literature of greater significance was beginning to develop at the same time. This literature, brought together and critically reviewed by von Senden, reflected the existence of a substantial population of individuals born with congenital cataracts that were subsequently surgically eliminated. This population lacked visual form experience early in life, and was of interest to von Senden primarily with regard to the question of the role of the various senses in the development of spatial perception. However, von Senden also noted the existence of apparently permanent, optically noncorrectable deficits in form vision, a finding that strongly implied some effect of early visual experience on visual system organization.

While significant for later work, the major impetus for research related to visual system plasticity during the earlier part of the 20th century turned out not to be the more general problem of trying to unravel the contributions of innate and environmental factors in perception but rather the more local problem of trying to account for what was increasingly recognized to be a high degree of organization in brain development itself. Many philosophers, psychologists, and biologists were already convinced that a major part of brain organization was innately determined. Ramon y Cajal and others had concluded that initial axonal outgrowth was not random but rather highly directed. Paul Weiss reported experimental studies implying that functional organization in the motor system was innately determined. However, Weiss also reported additional observations in tissue culture that led him to doubt that the controls on axonal outgrowth were sufficiently precise to account for the high degree of functional organization, and Karl Lashley reported findings suggesting that connection patterns were not in fact the critical feature determining brain function. It was in this context that a series of observations by Roger Sperry, beginning in the 1940s and extending into the 1960s, led to a more precise formulation of problems in visual system development (and nervous system development generally) and to a resulting change in the meaning of plasticity.

Sperry's observations began with studies of the recovery of visual orienting behavior associated with optic nerve regeneration in amphibians, and largely paralleled Weiss's earlier work on motor systems. Like Weiss, Sperry recognized that functional recovery implies the reestablishment of orderly functional relationships between the periphery and the central nervous system, in this case between the retina and visual centers in the brain. Also like Weiss, Sperry performed experiments to determine whether the reestablishment was attributable to a process of testing and refinement based on sensory experience. Sperry's finding that the recovered behavior in eye-rotated animals was permanently maladaptive persuaded most workers that experience-dependent adaptive shaping was less significant in accounting for visual system organization than a genetically based process of self-differentiation. Of at least equal importance for subsequent research was Sperry's recognition that the behavior, while maladaptive, was orderly and exactly that which would be expected if the ganglion cells of the rotated eye had reestablished their original connections in the brain. It was this finding which inclined Sperry, unlike Weiss and Lashley, to conceive of the problem of functional organization in terms of anatomical connection between neurons, and to propose the *chemoaffinity hypothesis* as the solution to the developmental problem. In essence, the hypothesis represented a return to earlier assertions that orderly connectivity resulted from orderly growth processes, and in particular from a refined differentiation of neurons that allows them to recognize and distinguish among possible targets. Anatomical, electrophysiological, and embryological findings during the 1960s provided support for the hypothesis and have clearly established that intercellular recognition processes represent a major determinant of neuronal connectivity patterns.

The second phase: Plasticity vs. specificity

During the period between the 1940s and the mid-1960s, the simplicity and apparent successes of the chemoaffinity hypothesis largely removed from center stage interest in the involvement of sensory experience in visual system development, to say nothing of interest in the more general problem of accounting for the adaptive character of visual system organization. The obvious behavioral and psychological reality that experience affects visual processing was largely ignored. So too were findings such as those indicating that while placement of rotating prisms in front of the eyes in humans led initially, as with eye rotations in frogs, to maladaptive behavior, the behavior, unlike that in frogs, was corrected with experience. These and similar observations were generally regarded as related to unknown higher level processes, and not as a serious challenge to the hypothesis that the basic connection patterns of the visual system were determined genetically by events in early development. The only serious challenges to the chemoaffinity hypothesis were observations suggesting that the targets of axons were not in fact so rigidly determined by early events, and it was to findings of this kind that the term plasticity referred during the next phase of research.

Three sets of findings during the 1960s and early 1970s epitomized visual system plasticity in this sense. The first was the finding that early visual deprivation has dramatic and permanent effects on the visual responsiveness of neurons in the mammalian visual cortex. The second was a series of observations suggesting that following various kinds of surgical intervention retinal ganglion cells in fish and amphibians would in fact form connections at abnormal locations. The third was the finding that removal of one eye early in life in mammals resulted in abnormal projections from the remaining eye. It

is of interest that only the last of these findings was actually an anatomical observation. The others were, however, presumed to closely reflect anatomical patterns of connections, and subsequent work has largely, though not completely, born this out. Of greater interest is that none of the three sets of findings, at least initially, were regarded as a challenge to the general notion of early, genetically based determination of connection patterns. The deprivation findings and related studies were interpreted not as evidence for an adaptively significant modifiability, but rather as evidence that a genetically based normal network could be disturbed by abnormal visual experience. The findings on retinal projections in fish and amphibians, and those on the effects of eye removal in mammals were interpreted as suggesting the existence of additional cellular mechanisms that could, instead of or in addition to intracellular recognition processes, produce the normal connection pattern.

This agnostic period of research, which continues to some extent today, was an enormously active one, and provided a substantial body of important description about the degree to which connection patterns could be altered by various sorts of experimental perturbations. The phenomenon of critical periods, that systems are more sensitive to perturbation at certain developmental times than others, was clearly documented. So too was the phenomenon of competition, the observation that the particular connections and even the growth and survival of one population of neurons, could be influenced by the presence or absence of other populations of neurons projecting to the same general location. A related phenomenon, that the terminal field of a given neuronal population has a tendency to expand if possible, was also established. Finally, enough information was gathered to make it clear electrical activity in general, and sensory experience in particular, can affect connection patterns, and hence to reawaken interest in their possible role in adaptive shaping of such patterns. More generally, research during this period sufficiently unsettled the prevailing view of a rigidly genetically determined connection pattern to encourage new inquiries into the possibility of functionally significant modifiability of the visual pathways.

The third phase: Plasticity as adaptively significant modifiability

Several lines of evidence, in addition to the finding that processes other than cellular recognition can influence connection patterns, have contributed to the current perspective that there is a substantial capacity for adaptively significant modifiability in the visual system. The most compelling, if not in general the most influential, has been the direct demonstration, primarily in fish and amphibians, that adaptively significant changes in connection patterns do in fact occur during individual lifetimes. The tectal terminals of retinal ganglion cells shift during growth, most probably due to the intrinsic expansion and competition phenomena mentioned earlier. Recent findings suggest that influences of electrical activity on terminal formation may also be involved. In amphibians, there is an additional dramatic change in the retinofugal projections, with an uncrossed retinofugal component first appearing during metamorphosis. The latter appears to reflect hormonal actions on the nervous system.

Direct evidence for successive, adaptively appropriate changes in connection patterns during individual lifetimes in mammals has yet to be obtained, probably because investigators of these species have been less inclined to identify and explore particular functional situations in which they might be expected to occur. On the other hand, studies of normal development have revealed that the initial connection patterns formed at a number of different locations in the visual pathways are more diffuse than those seen later, a finding widely interpreted as indicative of the existence of a potential for adaptively significant modification of connection patterns, at least during early developmental stages. Consistent with this are experimental observations in at least some cases indicating that surgical manipulations or alterations of visual experience can influence the connection pattern that emerges from the diffuse phase.

Studies specifically of the development of binocular organization have played an especially significant role in current perspectives on plasticity. Findings in the early 1970s triggered a reevaluation of the involvement of visual experience in mammalian cortical development, leading to the conclusion that visual experience plays an important role in creating the highly precise alignment of projections from the two eyes observed physiologically in cortical neurons. Studies on tectal binocularity in amphibians, appearing at about the same time, also implied an important involvement of visual experience in aligning projections from the two eyes. Findings in the two cases are largely parallel and represent an instance partially but not completely satisfying the definition of plasticity used early in the century, as well as the focus on anatomical organization that developed subsequently. Binocularity is partially but not entirely a reflection of adaptive shaping. Instead, early developmental events produce a rough alignment that can then, within limits, be refined by visual experience. The shaping is probably based not on a direct test of functional appropriateness but rather on an indirect criterion, such as synchrony of activity from the two eyes. The shaping process does at least to some degree reflect alterations in connection patterns, but there is reason to suspect that the anatomical correlates currently known may not fully account for the functional adjustments.

Future trends

The evolution of the meaning of plasticity reflects substantial progress in research on visual processing and on brain function generally. The modern understanding that there exists a variety of mechanisms by which adaptive adjustments may be brought about in the anatomical structures of the visual system is clinically significant and also helps to explain the remarkable success of the brain in dealing with complex information processing tasks. At the same time, it seems clear that a number of significant adaptive processes remain to be accounted for, and that as research is increasingly directed toward these further evolution of the meaning of plasticity is likely. Significant variations in visual behavior, for example, the adjustments of humans to inverting prisms, occur over time courses almost certainly too short to be accounted for by variations in anatomical connectivity of the kind explored in most of the studies currently regarded as directed at plasticity. Recent work on visually elicited orienting behaviors in primates and frogs suggests that the interpretation placed on signals in the visual pathways varies substantially depending on the character of contemporaneous signals in other pathways. It is likely that with further work in these areas, and on the older issue of the genesis of spatial perception, plasticity will come to mean more broadly ''the capacity to make appropriate adjustments in visual function,'' and that currently described phenomena related to alterability of anatomical structures will be seen as a subset of the broader category.

Further reading

Cowan WM, Fawcett JW, O'Leary DM, Stanfield B (1980): Regressive events in neurogenesis. *Science* 225:1258–1265

Easter SS (1986): The development and regeneration of the retinotectal projection. In: *Handbook of Physiology, Development of the Nervous System.* Cowan WM, Edwards JS, eds. Bethesda: American Physiological Society

Grobstein P (1987): On beyond neuronal specificity: Problems in going from cells to networks and networks to behavior. In: *Neural and Behavioral Development, Vol 3.* Shinkman P, ed. New York: Ablex

Sherman SM, Spear PD (1982): Organization of visual pathways in normal and visually deprived cats. *Physiol Rev* 62:738–855

Sperry RW (1965): Embryogenesis of behavioral nerve nets. In: *Organogenesis.* DeHaan RL, Ursprung H, eds. New York: Holt, Rinehart, and Winston

Visual Transduction

Gordon L. Fain and *Wayne L. Hubbell*

Figure 1A is a schematic representation of the salient structural features of the vertebrate rod cell. As indicated, the cell has two distinct anatomical regions, the inner and outer segments. The inner segment contains the subcellular organelles required for the usual metabolic processes of the cell and terminates in a synaptic foot. The outer segment is specialized for phototransduction and is densely packed with a highly ordered stack of flattened membrane saccules generally referred to as discs, the individual membranes of which contain the integral membrane protein rhodopsin in high concentration. The rims of the discs have an exceedingly small radius of curvature and are specialized structures with a composition distinctly different from the planar regions of the membrane. The adjacent membranes of a disc lie in close apposition, resulting in a very attenuated intradiscal spacing of only about 30 Å. The highly regular spacing between adjacent discs (approximately

150 Å) and between the disc rims and the plasma membrane of the outer segment is apparently achieved by filamentous structures that bridge the interdisc and disc-plasma membrane spaces. This cytoskeletal network is presumably responsible for the observed structural rigidity of the outer segment.

Although the disc and plasma membrane systems are structurally connected, they are functionally separate and in rods show no membrane continuity except at the base of the outer segment where a few new discs are in the process of formation by invagination of the plasma membrane. In the other sort of vertebrate photoreceptor, the cones, the discs are continuous with the plasma membrane, and the inside of the disc is open to the extracellular space. Despite the nearly crystalline appearance of the disc array, the membranes themselves are highly fluid and support a rapid rotational and translational diffusion of the rhodopsin molecule, providing for equal probabilities

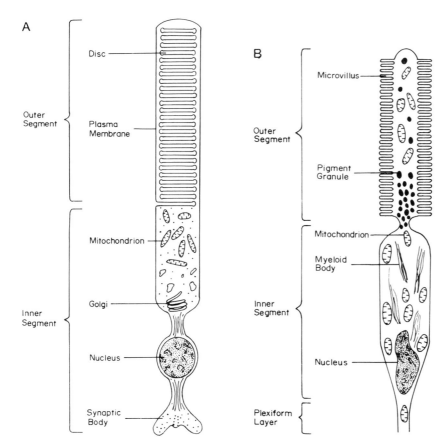

Figure 1. A. Schematic drawing of a bovine rod cell. The intra and interdiscal spacings are highly exaggerated for clarity. B. Schematic drawing of a squid photoreceptor cell. The average length of a microvillus is 1.1 μ in squid, and its average diameter is 0.1 μ. There are several hundred thousand microvilli per photoreceptor.

of photon capture for all polarizations of incident radiation.

Figure 1B shows the anatomy of a representative invertebrate photoreceptor cell, in this case the squid. The rhodopsin molecules are located in cylindrical microvillar structures which (as for the discs of cones) are continuous with the plasma membrane, and the rhodopsin molecules are rotationally restricted, providing for differential sensitivity to different polarizations of incident radiation.

The chromophoric group in both vertebrate and invertebrate rhodopsins is 11-*cis* retinal (except in freshwater fish, amphibians, and reptiles where 11-*cis* dehydroretinal as well as 11-*cis* retinal may be employed). The retinal is covalently attached to the protein through a protonated schiff-base linkage to lysine. The sole photochemical result of photon absorption by rhodopsin is the isomerization of the chromophore from the 11-*cis* to the all-*trans* form.

The amino acid sequence of the bovine rhodopsin molecule has recently been determined. Predictive methods based on hydrophobicity together with chemical information have allowed the construction of tentative molecular models. It appears likely that the molecule consists of seven transmembrane alpha helices with the carboxy-terminus at the disc membrane cytoplasmic surface and the amino-terminus at the intradiscal surface. The two carbohydrate chains on rhodopsin are linked to asparagine residues near the amino-terminus. The bulk of the molecular mass is located within the low dielectric region of the membrane. Light absorption has no significant effect on the secondary structure of the molecule, although subtle conformational changes in tertiary structure clearly occur.

The absorption of light by rhodopsin results in the closure of plasma membrane ionic channels in a highly amplified fashion. Since in rods rhodopsin is in the disc membrane and the channels are in the plasma membrane, these events must be mediated by an internal messenger system. This is probably also true for cones. It is generally agreed that the internal messenger is a low-molecular weight, diffusable substance whose activity is modulated by the absorption of light by rhodopsin. The identity of the messenger and the mechanism of its action are unknown, but there is strong evidence suggesting the involvement of Ca^{++} and cyclic guanosine monophosphate (cGMP).

Rod outer segments contain a substantial amount of Ca^{++} ion, on the order of one to two ions per rhodopsin molecule. If this Ca^{++} were distributed uniformly throughout the outer segment, it would amount to a concentration of 2.5–5 mM. However, the free cytoplasmic levels of Ca^{++} are less than micromolar, and it is likely that the majority of the outer segment Ca^{++} is localized within the intradiscal space where its concentration could be as high as 30 mM if none were surface bound. Light excitation of the photoreceptor causes an extrusion into the extracellular space of as many as 10^4 Ca^{++} per photolyzed rhodopsin on the time scale of the photoresponse, indicating an amplified release of the intradiscal stores of the ion. Research is aimed at quantifying the light-dependent redistribution of Ca^{++} and elucidating the mechanism of Ca^{++} mobilization or transport and the role of rhodopsin photolysis in its control.

Rod outer segments contain both cGMP and a cGMP phosphodiesterase (PDE) that is activated by photolyzed rhodopsin in a process mediated by a nucleotide binding protein variously referred to as G or transducin (Fig. 2). In the dark, G-protein contains a bound molecule of GDP. When a photolyzed rhodopsin molecule in the membrane (Rh*) encounters a G molecule, a complex is formed which catalyzes the exchange of the bound GDP for a GTP. Once the G_{GTP} complex is formed, it dissociates from Rh*, and the cycle is repeated, resulting

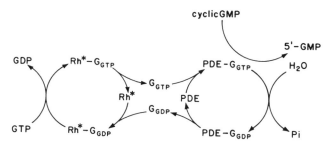

Figure 2. Cyclic nucleotide cascade of vertebrate rod photoreceptor. Rh*, photoactivated rhodopsin; G_{GTP} and G_{GDP}, activated G-protein complexes; PDE, phosphodiesterase.

in the formation of many G_{GTP} complexes per Rh*. G_{GTP} complexes encounter and activate PDE molecules by releasing an inhibitory subunit bound to PDE. Finally, the activated (PDE) hydrolyzes cGMP to GMP. G_{GTP} complexes become incompetent in activating PDE when the GTPase activity of G hydrolyzes the bound GTP to GDP to yield the dark state. The net result of this cycle is a light-stimulated, highly amplified hydrolysis of the cGMP in which a single photolyzed rhodopsin results in the hydrolysis of as many as 10^5 cGMP molecules. The operation of this cycle in the cytoplasm of the outer segment could certainly lead to a substantial reduction of the cGMP levels and a possible role for the nucleotide as a messenger. An important area of current research is to identify the target of cGMP action. Interestingly, this cyclic nucleotide cascade is strikingly similar to that which mediates the action of beta-adrenergic hormones.

In addition to exposing a binding site for G-protein, photolysis of rhodopsin exposes multiple sites near the carboxy-terminus susceptible to phosphorylation by an endogenous kinase. The role of the phosphorylation is uncertain, but it may be the mechanism whereby Rh* is terminated as an activator of the GDP-GTP exchange on G.

Invertebrate photoreceptors, such as in squid, also contain a G-protein that incorporates both GTP binding and hydrolysis functions that can be activated by interaction with photolyzed rhodopsin. Whether regulation of endogenous phosphodiesterase or cyclase activities results from activation of the G species is not yet resolved.

Whatever the exact mechanism of transduction, the end result is a change in the membrane potential of the photoreceptor. In most invertebrates, this is produced by an increase in conductance primarily to Na^+, which depolarizes the cell (see Fig. 3A). In vertebrates, on the other hand, the photoreceptors are depolarized in the dark. Unlike most neurons, vertebrate rods and cones have a large resting permeability to Na^+. Since this permeability is restricted to the outer segment of the cell, a large current enters the outer segment in darkness. The Na^+ current entering the outer segment is balanced by a K^+ current leaving the inner segment, and the Na^+ and K^+ activities are maintained by an abundant Na^+-K^+ activity located in the membrane of the inner segment (see Fig. 1A). This continual recycling of Na^+ and K^+ through the receptor may seem wasteful, but it probably serves the important function of biasing the dark resting membrane potential of rods and cones to a region of greater sensitivity for synaptic transmitter release. Light reduces the receptor Na^+ permeability, decreases the current entering the outer segment, and hyperpolarizes the membrane potential (see Fig. 3B).

Although the responses of vertebrate and invertebrate photo-

Figure 3. Electrical responses of photoreceptors to light. A. Intracellular voltage response of invertebrate photoreceptor, based on recordings from ventral eye of horseshoe crab *Limulus polyphemus*. B. Intracellular voltage response of vertebrate rod, based on recordings from toad *Bufo marinus*. Lower traces indicate duration of light stimuli. See text for explanation of arrow.

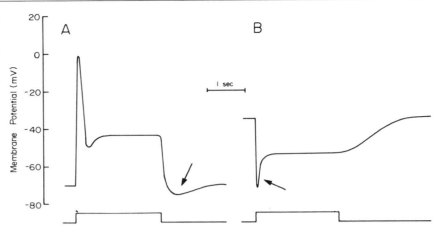

receptors differ in polarity, they nevertheless show several striking similarities. The reversal potentials for both range from +5 to +15. Under physiological conditions the light-dependent currents are carried primarily by Na+, but the light-dependent channels appear none the less to be nonselective in both vertebrates and invertebrates, admitting all the alkali cations and some divalent cations (in rods) or large organic cations like choline (in arthropods). The voltage dependence of the light-dependent conductance in the two groups also appears to be quite similar, the conductance increasing strongly at positive potentials (outwardly rectifying). The single channels have been reported to have a mean conductance of 25 pS in rods and of about 40pS in *Limulus polyphemus*.

Analysis of the waveform of the photoreceptor light response reveals that transduction in both vertebrates and invertebrates is a complex process, consisting of several stages from the absorption of a photon to the change in membrane potential. However, the exact role of the various biochemical changes described above is not yet known, and in particular, it is unclear how changes in the concentration of cyclic nucleotides, Ca^{++}, and other putative internal messengers produce the opening or closing of the light-dependent channels. In rods, injections of activated G-protein or of cGMP phosphodiesterase hyperpolarize the rod membrane potential, thus mimicking the light response. Furthermore, increases in rod cGMP levels produce membrane depolarization and slowing of the response waveform. Finally, cGMP on isolated patches of rod outer segment membrane has been shown to modulate a conductance similar to the light-dependent conductance. It therefore seems likely that the enzymatic cascade leading from activation of G-protein to the hydrolysis of cGMP (see Fig. 2) has some direct role in the generation of the light response. On the other hand, increases in intracellular Ca^{++} produce a clear decrease in the outer segment Na+ permeability and also hyperpolarize the rod membrane potential, but it is uncertain whether this is a direct effect on channels. In invertebrates (*Limulus polyphemus*), channels can be opened by injections of cGMP, Ca^{++}, and inositol 1,4,5-trisphosphate. Which if any of these directly produces the increase in Na+ permeability during the light response is unknown.

In addition to the light-dependent conductance, photoreceptors have a variety of voltage or calcium-dependent currents which in some cases contribute to the waveform of the light response. In rods, the most important of these is the so-called Cs^+-sensitive conductance (or gh), which has a reversal potential near -30 mV (close to the dark resting membrane potential) and is activated by membrane hyperpolarization. It closely resembles the gf of heart Purkinje fibers. An increase in this conductance during the light response depolarizes the cell and produces a pronounced sag in the voltage (Fig. 3B, **arrow**), thus preventing the cell from hyperpolarizing beyond the region of high sensitivity for synaptic transmitter release. In invertebrates there are voltage-dependent inward-going Na+ and Ca^{++} currents that generate one to two action potentials on the rising phase of the light response. There are also voltage-dependent $K+$ conductances that modify the falling phase of the waveform. At the termination of the response to bright light, there is a pronounced hyperpolarization (Fig. 3A, arrow), which is produced by an electrogenic Na^+-K^+ ATPase.

Recordings from receptors have revealed several of the basic features of phototransduction. The generation of the light response is extremely localized in both vertebrate and invertebrate receptors, spreading little from the site of photon absorption. The high sensitivity of photoreceptors indicates that the transduction process must have a large gain. In *Limulus polyphemus*, a single absorbed quantum produces a photocurrent of at least 2 nA, equivalent to the net movement of 10^8–10^9 Na+ and the opening of about 10^4 channels. Rods also respond to single quanta, though the quantal current is about three orders of magnitude smaller (about 10^{-12} amp). In cones, the sensitivity of transduction is even lower (about 10^{-14} amp per quantum), suggesting possible differences in the mechanism of response generation in the two kinds of vertebrate receptors.

When photoreceptors are exposed to continuous light, their sensitivity decreases. The brighter the light, the larger the decrease in sensitivity. This process, called light adaptation, extends the range of illuminations over which photoreceptors are capable of responding. It is a basic feature of phototransduction in most organisms. In the rods of poikilotherms, light adaptation begins in very dim illumination, and the absorption of only a few photons per rod is enough to produce a significant change in sensitivity. Since rods have 1000–2000 discs (see Fig. 1A), isomerization of the photopigment in only a small percentage of the discs must be able to alter the sensitivity of transduction in the whole of the rod. In cones, much brighter lights are necessary before significant changes in sensitivity occur. In bright illumination, the decrease in sensitivity in most receptors is approximately proportional to the intensity of the continuous background light (Weber-Fechner law) and extends over a range of at least 4 orders of magnitude. An exception to this is the mammalian rod, which adapts over a much more restricted range.

Some properties of light adaptation can be inferred from changes in the light response waveform in the presence of continuous illumination. In vertebrates, background light has no effect on the latency or initial time course of the receptor response. This suggests that adaptation does not alter the initial steps in transduction up to and including the production of the excitatory messenger. Background light does produce a dramatic quickening of the time course of response decay, as if the lifetime of the excitatory messenger (or of its effect on the Na^+ channels) were greatly shortened. In invertebrates (principally *Limulus polyphemus*), the effects of background light can be mimicked by the intracellular injection of Ca^{++} and prevented by injection of Ca buffers like EGTA. These observations indicate that Ca^{++} may have some role in mediating adaptation in invertebrates.

After exposure to bright light, the sensitivity of photoreceptors increases back to its initial value in the dark. This process, called dark adaptation, is complex and appears to consist of several phases with different time courses. It is probably caused by the gradual recovery of membrane conductance, ion gradients, disc Ca^{++} stores, enzyme activities, and the concentrations of metabolites to their dark-adapted levels. In vertebrate photoreceptors, there is a slow recovery phase with approximately the same time course as the regeneration of the photopigment. This phase of dark adaptation is much slower in rods than in cones, perhaps as a result of differences in the mechanisms of pigment regeneration in the two photoreceptors.

Further reading

Fain G, Lisman J (1981): Membrane conductors in photoreceptors. *Proc Biophys Mol Biol* 37:91–147

Hargrave P (1982): Rhodopsin chemistry, structure and topography. In: *Progress in Retinal Research, Vol 1*, Osbourne N, Chader G, eds. New York: Pergamon Press

Kuhn H (1984) Interactions between photoexcited rhodopsin and light-activated enzymes in rods. In: *Progress in Retinal Research, Vol 3*, Osbourne N, Chader G, eds. New York: Pergamon Press

Miller W (1981): *Current Topics in Membranes and Transport, Vol 15*. New York: Academic Press

Stryer L (1986): Cyclic GMP cascade of vision. *Ann Rev Neurosci.* 9:87–119

Visual-Vestibular Interaction

Volker Henn

The sense of motion uses information from different sensory receptor organs. For humans, vestibular inputs from the inner ear and the visual system are the most important. The experience of a unique sense of motion independent of the sensory system from which the information comes requires that these different messages converge. The site and neuronal mechanism of this convergence have been widely investigated in monkeys. (Anatomical and behavioral studies indicate that mechanisms in humans are similar.)

The first convergence of vestibular and visual input takes place in the vestibular nuclei, only one synapse away from the hair cells in the labyrinths (see Fig. 1). Figure 2 shows a typical cell in the vestibular nuclei with a resting discharge of 30 imp/sec which receives input from the horizontal semicircular canal. During angular acceleration in the horizontal plane, its activity increases and during constant velocity rotation, it approaches the level of spontaneous activity with a characteristic time constant (Fig. 2). If the visual surround is rotated around the stationary animal, the cell's activity increases and keeps its activity until all motion ceases. If the animal is rotated in the light, the activity induced by labyrinthine and visual stimulation combines to induce activity that, over a large range, is proportional to actual rotational velocity. This is the typical activity found in response to vestibular and visual stimuli for all cells in the vestibular nuclei. In a quantitative way there are differences in sensitivity and working range.

For the visual and labyrinthine motion information to combine, it must be coded in the same dimension. Directions are determined by the three planes of semicircular canals. As the vestibular nerve connects to three different classes of cells in the nuclei, these canal-specific planes are maintained. Activity related to visual stimulation is proportional to the velocity of the stimulus. Labyrinthine activity induced by angular acceleration is partially integrated mechanically by the cupula and neuronally in the vestibular nuclei, so that it also represents a velocity signal over a wide range of frequencies.

One can postulate that activity from the otoliths and the visual system that conveys information about linear motion combines in a similar way, but this has not been investigated in detail.

Further sites of interaction between visual and vestibular inputs are necessary because the vestibular system simultaneously serves different purposes—conveying an accurate sense of motion, moving the eyes in order to stabilize vision during head movement, and stabilizing posture. During the same head movement, we might have compensatory eye movements, or we might want to suppress them because we foveate on a moving target. The labyrinthine activity will be the same during the two movements, giving rise to the same sensation of movement. In the first case this activity will be used to induce compensatory eye movements; in the second case this activity projecting to the oculomotor system has to be canceled or suppressed. This is one of the functions of the flocculus. It has reciprocal connections with the vestibular nuclei and receives visual input through mossy and climbing fibers. Based

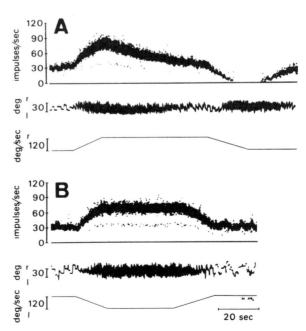

Figure 2. Activity of a neuron in the vestibular nuclei of a monkey in response to vestibular stimulation (A, angular acceleration in darkness), and visual stimulation (B, rotation of an optokinetic cylinder around the stationary animal). From the top down, instantaneous neuronal frequency, horizontal eye position, and stimulus velocity. From Waespe and Henn (1977).

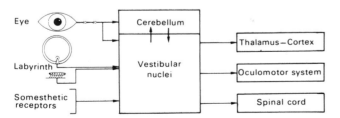

Figure 1. Diagram of how information about motion from different receptor systems converge upon the vestibular nuclei and give off three distinct pathways apart from a dense reciprocal connection with the floccular-nodular lobe of the cerebellum.

on various studies, the function of the flocculus is to enhance or reduce eye velocity to adjust it to the velocity of the visual target.

In a similar interactive way inputs combine to produce somatic motor responses (mediated via the vestibulospinal tract among others) to stabilize posture.

The vestibular nuclei project to the thalamus and cortex, a necessary input for all conscious experience. As the information from individual sensory systems is combined, the unique message from the individual sense loses its identity. We cannot discriminate the individual inputs to the vestibular nuclei and so we experience but one unique sense of self-motion.

Further reading

Henn V, Cohen B, Young LR (1980): Visual-vestibular interaction in motion perception and the generation of nystagmus. *Neurosci Res Prog Bull* 18:457–651

Waespe W, Henn V (1977): Neuronal activity in the vestibular nuclei of the alert monkey during vestibular and optokinetic stimulation. *Exp Brain Res* 27:523–538

Contributors

John Allman Professor of Biology, California Institute of Technology, Pasadena, California 91125, U.S.A.

John C. Armington Department of Psychology, Northeastern University, Boston, Massachusetts 02115, U.S.A.

Emilio Bizzi Department of Brain and Cognitive Sciences, Massachusetts Institute of Technology, Cambridge, Massachusetts 02139, U.S.A.

G.S. Brindley Medical Research Council, Neurological Prostheses Unit, Institute of Psychiatry, De Crespigny Park, London SE5, England

Kao Liang Chow Department of Neurology, Stanford University, School of Medicine, Palo Alto, California 94304, U.S.A.

Max Cynader Killam Research Professor, Fellow, Canadian Institute for Advanced Research, Departments of Psychology, Physiology and Biophysics, Dalhousie University, Halifax, Nova Scotia, B3H 4J1, Canada

Nigel W. Daw Department of Cell Biology and Physiology, Washington University Medical School, St. Louis, Missouri 63110, U.S.A.

John E. Dowling Department of Cellular and Developmental Biology, Harvard University, Cambridge, Massachusetts 02138, U.S.A.

Mark Wm. Dubin Professor, Department of Molecular, Cellular, and Developmental Biology, University of Colorado, Boulder, Colorado 80309-0347, U.S.A.

Gordon L. Fain Department of Ophthalmology, Jules Stein Eye Institute, University of California, Los Angeles School of Medicine, Los Angeles, CA 90024, U.S.A.

John P. Frisby AI Vision Research Unit, University of Sheffield, Sheffield S10 2TN, United Kingdom

James P. Gaska Department of Neurology, University of Massachussetts Medical School, Worcester, Massachusetts 01605, U.S.A.

Reuben S. Gellman Laboratory of Sensorimotor Research, National Eye Institute, National Institutes of Health, Bethesda, Maryland 20205, U.S.A.

Paul Grobstein Department of Biology, Bryn Mawr College, Bryn Mawr, Pennsylvania 19010, U.S.A.

Lewis O. Harvey, Jr. Department of Psychology, University of Colorado, Boulder, Colorado 80309-0345, U.S.A.

Richard Held Professor of Experimental Psychology, Head, Department of Psychology, Massachusetts Institute of Technology, Cambridge, Massachusetts 02139, U.S.A.

Volker Henn Professor of Neurology, Neurology Department, University Hospital, CH-8081 Zürich, Switzerland

Wayne L. Hubbell Department of Ophthalmology, and Department of Chemistry and Biochemistry, Jules Stein Eye Institute, University of California, Los Angeles School of Medicine, Los Angeles, CA 90024, U.S.A.

Howard C. Hughes Department of Psychology, Dartmouth College, Hanover, New Hampshire 03755, U.S.A.

Leo M. Hurvich Department of Psychology, and Institute of Neurological Sciences, University of Pennsylvania, Philadelphia 19104, U.S.A.

David J. Ingle Department of Physiology, University of Connecticut, Storrs, Connecticut 06268, U.S.A.

Masao Ito Professor, Department of Physiology, Faculty of Medicine, University of Tokyo, Tokyo 113, Japan

Bela Julesz AT&T Bell Laboratories, Murray Hill, New Jersey 07974, U.S.A.

Marcel Kinsbourne Eunice Kennedy Shriver Center, Waltham, Massachusetts 02254, U.S.A., and Harvard Medical School, Boston, Massachusetts 02115, U.S.A.

Kuno Kirschfeld Max-Planck-Institut für Biologische Kybernetik, D-7400 Tübingen 1, Federal Republic of Germany

Christof Koch Division of Biology and Engineering, California Institute of Technology, Pasadena, California 91125, U.S.A.

Stephen M. Kosslyn Department of Psychology, Harvard University, Cambridge, Massachusetts 02138, U.S.A.

Edwin H. Land The Rowland Institute for Science, Cambridge, Massachusetts 02142, U.S.A.

Theodore Lawwill Professor and Chairman, Department of Ophthalmology, University of Kansas Medical Center, Kansas City, Kansas 66103, U.S.A.

Eduardo R. Macagno Department of Biological Sciences, Columbia University, New York, New York 10027, U.S.A.

Ian A. Meinertzhagen Life Sciences Centre, Dalhousie University, Halifax, Nova Scotia, B3H 4JI, Canada

Frederick A. Miles Laboratory of Sensorimotor Research, National Eye Institute, National Institutes of Health, Bethesda, Maryland 20205, U.S.A.

Teruya Ohtsuka Department of Information Physiology, National Institute for Physiological Sciences, Okazaki 444, Japan

Pedro Pasik Professor of Neurology and Anatomy, Mount Sinai School of Medicine of the City University of New York, New York, New York 10029, U.S.A.

Tauba Pasik Professor of Neurology, Mount Sinai School of Medicine of the City University of New York, New York, New York 10029, U.S.A.

Daniel A. Pollen Department of Neurology, University of Massachusetts Medical School, Worcester, Massachusetts 01605, U.S.A.

Ernst Pöppel Institut für Medizinische Psychologie, Ludwig-Maximilians-Universität, D-8000 München 2, Federal Republic of Germany

Dianna A. Redburn University of Texas Medical School, Houston, Texas 77025, U.S.A.

Werner Reichardt Max-Planck-Institut für Biologische Kybernetik, D-7400 Tübingen 1, Federal Republic of Germany

Peter H. Schiller   Department of Brain and Cognitive Sciences, Massachusetts Institute of Technology, Cambridge, Massachusetts 02139, U.S.A.

S.C. Sharma   Department of Ophthalmology and Anatomy, New York Medical College, Valhalla, New York 10595, U.S.A.

Carla J. Shatz   Department of Neurobiology, Stanford University School of Medicine, Stanford, California 94305, U.S.A.

James M. Sprague   Department of Anatomy and Institute of Neurological Sciences, University of Pennsylvania School of Medicine, Philadelphia, Pennsylvania 19104, U.S.A.

Shimon Ullman   Department of Brain and Cognitive Sciences and the Artificial Intelligence Laboratory, Massachusetts Institute of Technology, Cambridge, Massachusetts 02139, U.S.A., and Department of Applied Mathematics, The Weizmann Institute, Rehovot, Israel

David C. Van Essen   Biology Division, California Institute of Technology, Pasadena, California 91125, U.S.A.

Christopher Walsh   Committee on Neurobiology and Pritzker School of Medicine, University of Chicago, Chicago, Illinois 60637, U.S.A., and Neurology Service, Massachusetts General Hospital, Boston, Massachusetts 02114, U.S.A.

Jeremy M. Wolfe   Department of Brain and Cognitive Sciences, Massachusetts Institute of Technology, Cambridge, Massachusetts 02139, U.S.A.